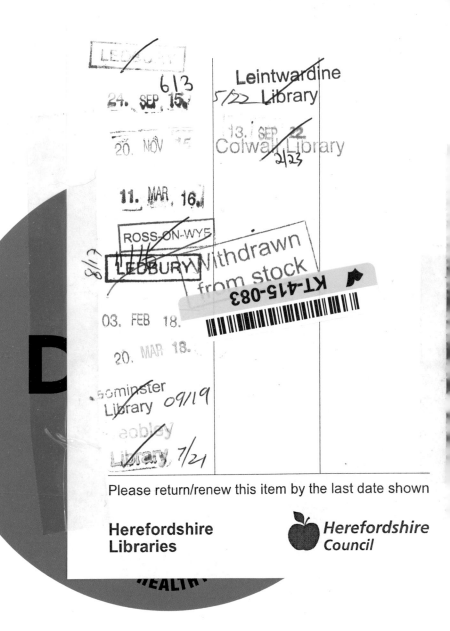

14 plans to combat the effects of modern life

DETOX

HELEN FOSTER

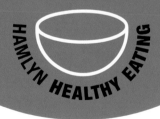

HAMLYN HEALTHY EATING

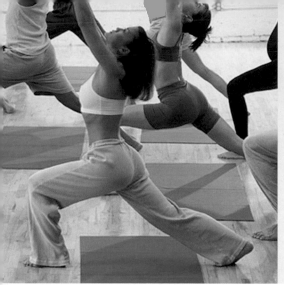

Safety Note
This book should not be considered a replacement for professional medical treatment; a physician should be consulted in all matters relating to health, particularly in respect of pregnancy and any other symptoms which may require diagnosis or medical attention. While the advice and information in this book is believed to be accurate, and the step-by-step exercises devised to avoid strain, neither the author nor the publisher can accept any legal responsibility for any injury or illness sustained while following the treatments and diet plans.

An Hachette UK Company
www.hachette.co.uk

First published in Great Britain in 2003 by Hamlyn,
a division of Octopus Publishing Group Ltd,
Endeavour House, 189 Shaftesbury Avenue,
London WC2H 8JY
www.octopusbooks.co.uk

Revised editions 2004, 2009

This edition published in 2015

This material was previously published as *Detox Solutions*.

Helen Foster asserts the moral right to be identified as the author of this work.

ISBN 978-0-600-63032-6

A CIP catalogue record for this book is available from the British Library

Printed and bound in China

10 9 8 7 6 5 4 3 2 1

introduction 6

contents

- what are toxins? 8
- how the body detoxes naturally 11
- when toxins build up 12
- diet and detox 15
- exercise and detox 20

- external detoxing 28
- using aromatherapy 34
- using supplements 38
- side-effects 41

detoxing: the plans 42
- using the plans 43
- lighten-up plan 44
- anti-pollution plan 48
- decaf plan 56
- sugar-busting plan 60
- stress-busting plan 66
- pre-party plan 74
- post-party hangover plan 78

- stop smoking plan 82
- energizing plan 90
- good health plan 96
- weight-loss plan 100
- beauty-boosting plan 108
- anti-cellulite plan 114
- live longer plan 121

index 126

acknowledgements 128

introduction

Detox – short for 'detoxification' – is possibly the biggest health topic of the 21st century. Studies have shown that we're feeling sicker and lower in energy than ever before. According to UK health magazine, *Top Santé*, 51 per cent of British women are tired all the time. Other research from the government-run Office of National Statistics has shown that British workers are taking 300,000 more sick days a year, with women suffering more than men. In the USA, a nationwide survey from the National Sleep Foundation showed that 63 million people, one-third of the population, are exhausted during the day, and 22 million working days a year are lost due to the increased incidence of colds alone.

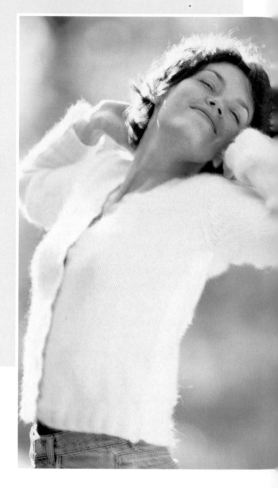

We know we have a problem and we know what we believe to be the reason: we are filling our bodies with toxins. These include the caffeine that we use to fuel our energy deficit, the fumes we breathe in trying to get from A to B in the rush hour, the junk food we eat because we're too tired to cook and the alcohol we drink trying to tackle stress. The result is that most of us have tried, at some point, to detox our bodies in some way. We've tried giving up coffee for a week, or living on grapes for the weekend. We've rubbed in lotions, drunk potions and done things with hard-bristled brushes that left our skin rubbed raw for weeks. But nothing seems to work. Why?

TOXIC OVERLOAD
The reason is that what most people understand as 'detoxing' simply doesn't work. You can't atone for a year's worth of toxic overload by eating grapes or raw food for a weekend. The body just isn't designed that way. We are exposed to an enormous toxin load – each year, the population of the UK alone consumes:

- 200 million alcoholic drinks
- 83 billion cigarettes
- 1 million tonnes of pesticides on food.

We are exposed to up to 5,000 new chemicals a year, and even the average beauty regime exposes us to up to 150 potentially toxic ingredients on a daily basis. The result is that the body gets overwhelmed and can't cope.

A NEW APPROACH

But we are not defenceless. There is an approach to detoxing your body, described in this book, that will make an efficient and long-term difference to your health and the way you feel. This book works with your body to fight against toxic attack. You'll still have to alter your diet to cleanse your system, but you'll work with foods and other elements to help reinforce your natural detox processes. This means that when you expose your body to toxins it will be able to process them more effectively.

The approach accepts that exposure is inevitable. It realizes that you're human, life is harder than it's ever been before, cars are going to belch pollution, ready meals exist and that sometimes it's fun to go out and drink too much. Rather than telling you that all toxins are evil and that you should avoid them at all costs, this book will show you how to tackle toxins so they cause less damage; or, should you decide you want to eliminate them completely, how to do so without losing your mind or your ability to live a normal life. It will give you control over your body, control that modern life often takes away. It will give you strength, energy and the power to be at your best.

So what are you waiting for? It's time to start detoxing!

HOW TO USE THIS BOOK

The first part of this book provides basic knowledge on how to strengthen your detox system. By using the advice on these pages alone, and integrating the recommended foods, supplements, exercise and massage into your daily life, you can deal generally with toxic overload and make your body function more effectively. The second part contains 14 tailor-made plans that help tackle specific toxins or related problems that might be concerning you. For example, maybe Christmas or your birthday is coming up, and you know you're going to drink too much but you hate the way that makes you feel. By using the Pre-party Plan (see page 74), you can minimize those unpleasant feelings. Maybe you're a smoker who wants to give up, but thinks it'll be too hard. By following the advice in the Stop Smoking Plan (see page 82), you can use your body's natural system of elimination to cut your cravings and make the process easier.

what are toxins?

One dictionary defines a toxin as 'a poisonous substance of plant or animal origin' – ingest one of those and you could be in for some seriously sick-making effects, if not death. However, when most of us use the word 'toxin', we don't mean such things. Instead we mean substances we believe are bad for us, such as caffeine, nicotine, alcohol and perhaps red meat. While it's true that these can be toxic for our body in certain doses, they are not the only things we should be thinking about. So, to get you started on learning how to help make your body toxin-free, here's what you may need to be cutting down on – and why.

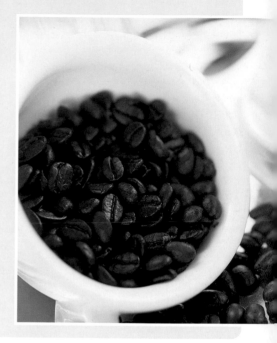

ALCOHOL

It's one of the toxins most of us worry about, but alcohol in small doses is actually harmless to the body. In fact, studies show that people who have one or two drinks a day are healthier and live longer than teetotallers. However, if you drink more than two a day this good news quickly becomes bad. Regularly drinking this amount can increase the risk of certain cancers and strokes, while binge drinking (defined as having more than four drinks in one day) can attack major organs, brain cells and vision. Still, most of us will find that three drinks in one evening is enough to ensure that we will have some level of hangover the next day.

CAFFEINE

We often hear people, ourselves included, say they must give up caffeine. But must we really give it up? While many of us think caffeine is a major toxin, the truth is there are no major health effects reported if you take in less than around 600mg a day (roughly six cups of coffee). In some people, however, minor health effects do occur at lower levels than this. As little as 350mg has been shown to lower concentration and energy levels, and research from Duke University in the USA has found that people whose intake is regularly greater than 400mg a day actually produce higher levels of stress hormones than those who consume less caffeine. Knowing how much you yourself consume can therefore be a valuable part of detoxing.

NICOTINE

From the ingredients used in cigarettes (and other smoking materials) and the reactions that occur when they are burned, you can take in 4,000 types of particle with every puff – many of them harmful. You will inhale poisons such as lead, arsenic and cyanide, and even in minute doses these don't do your body any good. You will also breathe in carbon monoxide, which starves the body of oxygen. Furthermore, during smoking your body produces chemicals, called nitrosamines, that cause cancer in practically everything they touch. If there's one vital step you can take to detox your body, it's to give up smoking.

PESTICIDES

It's estimated that the average person in the UK swallows around 4.5 litres (1 gallon) of pesticides each year in the food they consume. But, according to pressure group PAN UK, British people also expose themselves to over 4,306 tonnes of pesticides in their own homes through the use of insecticides, garden products and insect sprays. Other developed countries have similar statistics. Exactly what effects pesticides have on the body is still not understood, but fatigue, allergies, skin irritation and, at the most severe end of the spectrum, some forms of cancer have been linked to high exposure levels. Whether we ever reach such high levels in normal life is a matter of huge debate, but one thing is known – your body finds it very hard to detox pesticides naturally. Reducing exposure to them is therefore potentially more important than trying to eliminate them through strict diets.

FOOD INTOLERANCES

Can't lose weight? Fed up with the size of your stomach? Food intolerances could be the cause. These occur when the body loses the ability to digest a food properly. This results in the food staying in the system longer than it should. It then ferments, which allows toxins to be reabsorbed into the system. Intolerances have been linked to a head-to-toe map of symptoms, including headache, skin problems, weight gain, fluid retention, and even up to 65 per cent of cases of irritable bowel syndrome.

Intolerances develop when you are over-exposed to a food, which may explain why the two most common intolerances are wheat and dairy products, the staple foods of most of our diets since childhood.

One misunderstanding about food intolerance, though, is that once you find out you're intolerant to a food you can never eat it again. The good news, if you can't think of life without crusty French bread or a big plate of pasta, is that this is simply not true.

POLLUTANTS

Whether in the form of chemicals, hormones or heavy metals (like lead, mercury or aluminium), pollutants are creeping into all our lives. They may come from the air around us or from products we use in the home, or they may have found their way into our food through the soil or water. Pollutants can be very harmful to our systems. At the simplest level, research from the Children's Health Study in the USA has shown that on days when air pollution is at its highest, the rates of respiratory problems like sore throats and

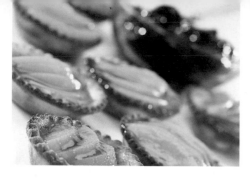

coughs in children increase. Pollutants are also a major cause of the harmful compounds called free radicals. These are unstable molecules that attack healthy cells in the body, creating damage. Free radicals have been linked to a host of problems, ranging from wrinkling of the skin to heart disease. The good news is that there has been a huge amount of research into the effects pollutants have on our bodies.

SATURATED (AND OTHER BAD) FATS

Detox purists will tell you that red meat is a toxin, because it's hard for the body to digest and therefore causes toxic build-up in the colon. It's even said that up to 2.2–4.5kg (5–10lb) of our body weight could be putrefied meat left in our colons. As yet, this has not been scientifically proven, so you can decide for yourself whether or not it's a good enough reason for you to cut red meat out of your diet.

What is true, however, is that many red meats (as well as a whole host of other foods such as full-fat dairy products, margarine and butter, cakes, biscuits and pastries) are high in saturated fat. This is bad news for your body, since the fats found in food need to be processed through the liver, and if it's doing this it can't spend as much time tackling true toxins like pesticides. What's more, saturated and other bad fats, such as trans fats or hydrogenated fats, increase the level of free radicals in the body.

However, even taking all of this into consideration, not all fat is bad – even the American Heart Association says that consuming up to 20g (¾oz) of saturated fat a day causes no harm to your body.

SUGAR

When most of us look at why sugar can be bad for us, we look at its effects on our waistline or teeth – but there's a bit more to it than that. When researchers at New York State University in Buffalo, USA, recently studied which foods produced the highest intake of free radicals in the body, sugar scored top. Within two hours of eating 300kcals of sugar (the equivalent of a can of fizzy drink and some chocolate), the number of free radicals increased by 140 per cent. Sugar also increases the levels of so-called 'bad' bacteria in the bowel, which can boost fermentation and increase the risk of more dangerous toxins being reabsorbed. For ultimate health, the US Department of Agriculture says we shouldn't eat more than 40g (1½oz) of sugar a day.

STRESS

You may not think of it as a toxin because stress isn't something you ingest (and it's probably not as dangerous as cigarettes) but it is still toxic to your body. When we get stressed, we produce a variety of chemicals in the body that put our system on alert. Our blood pressure increases and circulation speeds up, helping more dangerous toxins to circulate more freely throughout the system. When you become stressed, you're more likely to indulge in other toxins like alcohol, cigarettes and sugary or fatty comfort foods. Beating stress is an important part of detox – and it's also one of the nicest. No one has ever encountered a relaxation method they didn't like.

how the body detoxes naturally

The first thing you need to know about detoxing is that your body actually has a whole detox system of its own. It has to, otherwise it would become poisoned by natural toxins, including waste products from food, dead bacteria and debris from the millions of new cells produced each day. To appreciate how the detox plans work, you need to understand the basics of this system.

THE LIVER

Food is processed in the stomach and the small intestine. Useful products are absorbed and waste products sent to the detox system. Seventy-five per cent of these pass through the liver, where harmful toxins, which are not water-soluble, are neutralized by natural enzymes, so they become water-soluble, and are passed to the kidneys or bowel for excretion.

FAT STORES

If the liver is overwhelmed by toxins, it can't process them. So, instead the body pushes the toxins into the fat stores, where they do less damage.

THE KIDNEYS

The kidneys filter the blood, removing excess water and water-soluble toxins, that are then passed out in the urine.

THE SKIN

The skin, the largest organ of the body, also has a role to play in detox. Like the liver, the skin produces enzymes that make some of the toxins entering through it water-soluble.

These pass into the bloodstream and are excreted in urine or in sweat. Sweating also draws other toxins from the bloodstream.

THE LUNGS

The lungs remove carbon dioxide from the body and contain low levels of antioxidants, which neutralize free radicals. They also convert some toxins into water-soluble substances that can be exhaled.

THE LYMPHATIC SYSTEM

This series of tiny vessels runs into all areas of the body and transport nutrients in a fluid known as lymph. The lymphatic system is important in detox because it removes waste produced by the body; it's also a vital part of the body's immune system.

THE BOWEL

Harmful ingredients from the stomach are filtered out here and sent to the liver for processing. The bowel's main role is to excrete processed toxins in the faeces. If the bowel's function is sluggish, the faeces linger there and toxins can actually be reabsorbed into the bloodstream.

when toxins build up

When the body's natural detox system is working well, it can function at full power. However, if any one part of the system breaks down, toxins will not be eradicated, and will start to build up in the body. For example, the most simple (and probably most commonly experienced) sign of this is a hangover. If you exceed the amount of alcohol your body can process in one go, it starts to build up and effectively poisons the body, causing symptoms such as nausea, headache and an upset stomach. Once the body has had a chance to eliminate the alcohol, however, the symptoms begin to disperse.

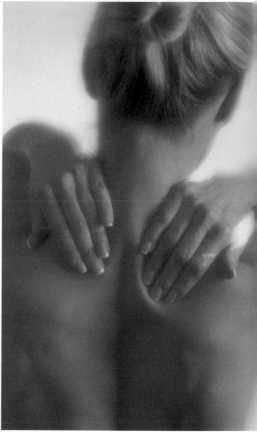

Now imagine this happening on a larger scale. If not removed effectively from the body, toxins can build up, stressing every system in our body and leading to problems like low energy, poor immunity, bad skin, cellulite, weight gain and even arthritis.

This outcome is what detoxing tries to tackle. The theory is, that if toxic overload doesn't happen in the first place, internal poisoning has no chance to occur either. By reducing your exposure to toxins, you can help take pressure off the body's natural detox system and allow it to deal

with those built-up toxins. It's a great idea but the problem is that, up until now, most of us have been doing it wrong.

WHY TRADITIONAL DETOX DOESN'T WORK
Last time you detoxed, what did you do? Chances are you will have cut out all toxin-forming foods, living on just fruit and vegetables for a few days, or perhaps you

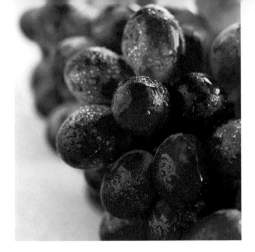

fibre, you're more likely to be constipated. During such a diet, the truth may be that you were actually plugging up another major elimination route.

CAN TRADITIONAL DETOX ACTUALLY HARM?

The scariest fact about strict detoxes comes from some Canadian research. Most of us carry out detox procedures because we're trying to tackle those mini-toxins that we inflict on our body every day – things like alcohol, red meat and caffeine – but by starving our bodies we may be releasing real toxins into the body. The reason for this is that starvation changes the way that we can produce energy.

Normally we use carbohydrates that are stored in the blood or muscles to give us our energy. However, after fasting for a day or so these stores are exhausted, so you're forced to get energy from your fat stores. Now, as explained earlier, if the body can't handle a toxin, it pushes it into the fat stores where it's safe – that is until those stores get broken down and the toxins are released into the bloodstream. While this may seem to prove the whole detox theory, what the Canadian researchers (from Quebec's Laval University) found was that once the chemicals they were investigating were released they didn't disappear. In fact, levels of them rose as the diets went on – it was as if the body simply didn't know how to handle them.

went on a juice fast. Doing this actually works against the way your body detoxes naturally. Common forms of detox may reduce the toxins that we take in, but they are also very low in calories. Also, when we fast in this way, the metabolic rate (the speed at which our body works) slows down by at least 10 per cent, and by even more as the fast continues. It only takes two days for this to happen, and it affects every process within the body, including that of waste removal – this is one of the processes that you want to make sure works thoroughly and effectively in order to get rid of the toxins in your body.

Therefore, on traditional detox plans, you could actually be eliminating toxins at a slower rate than normal. This slowing of the metabolism through such a detox will also lower your body temperature and, as it happens, reduce the amount you sweat – thereby cutting off another one of your major detox routes. To make things even worse, if you went on a juice diet you probably took all the fibre out of the healthy fruits and vegetables you were eating as you juiced them (unless you used a masticating juicer). This is a major problem, since the presence of fibre in the bowel stimulates it to work; if there's no

'On traditional detox plans, you could actually be eliminating toxins at a slower rate than normal.'

13

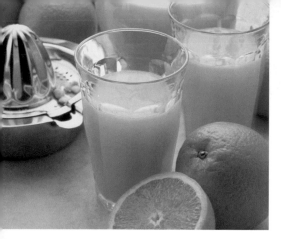

HELPING DETOX TO WORK

Reading all this, you're probably wondering why you have bought this book. If detoxing doesn't work, why has this book been written? There are two simple reasons.

The first is that detoxes – even traditional ones – do achieve something. A good detox diet focuses your mind on eating healthily and helps you reassess your relationship with foods that can sometimes be bad for you. For example, by giving up coffee for a week, you become less dependent on it to wake you up, and your natural energy becomes more balanced. By cutting out alcohol you remember how good it felt not to have a hangover, and you realize you can get through stressful situations without a glass of wine. By lowering your intake of sugar, you prevent the peaks and troughs in blood-sugar levels that can leave you fatigued and needing more sweet stuff to boost your energy. You also re-educate your tastebuds, making you less dependent on the 'bad foods', and in turn this helps to dramatically reduce the toxic load that your body is under.

The second reason is that the detox advice and plans in this book are not of the traditional variety. They not only harness all the positive benefits just described, but also do a great deal more.

WORKING WITH THE BODY

Rather than working against the natural process that your body uses to detox, the suggested solutions and plans in this book are designed to enhance it. They do this in two ways. First, like traditional detox programmes, they show you how to limit the amount of toxins you are exposed to, which reduces pressure on your detox system. However, you can do this without having to starve, which means your system can get to work. Second, the solutions work more effectively because the aim is to strengthen your natural detox system. This approach will enable you to:

• Increase production of the natural enzymes that your liver, skin and lungs use to neutralize harmful toxins, making it less likely that your body will suffer from toxic overload.

• Put in place defence mechanisms to neutralize harmful compounds that toxins bring into the body, reducing the damage they can cause.

• Boost blood flow around the system, which ensures that toxins are removed faster and more effectively.

• Strengthen the power of the skin and lungs to detox more effectively.

• Create a healthy digestive system, as well as ensuring the fast and effective removal of toxins.

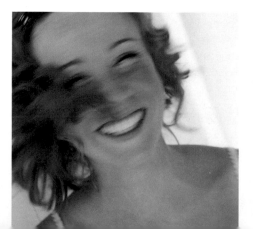

diet and detox

What you eat is the first line of defence against toxic attack. By controlling what goes into your mouth, you have the power to reduce a huge number of the toxins that could otherwise enter your body. This traditionally means giving up coffee, bread, milk, alcohol and red meat completely. If you want to do this, fine; but if giving up your morning coffee stops you detoxing your body in other ways, why bother? It's no fun and it's also unnecessary. As already mentioned, scientific evidence has shown that your body can tolerate one to two alcoholic drinks a day with no health problems and can easily deal with up to three cups of coffee a day with out adverse effects.

You may be surprised to learn this but your body can even tackle around 20g (¾oz) of saturated fat a day (the amount found in a 75g (3oz) serving of any lean red meat) with no health problems. If you are not intolerant to them, eating wheat and dairy foods will also have no ill effects. Therefore, despite their 'toxic' reputation, there's no reason why these foods shouldn't be part of your life – so long as you don't exceed those limits. What is important is reducing serious pollutants like pesticides, hormones and heavy metals.

REDUCING TOXIN INTAKE

In an ideal world, we would eat all organic food and get our eggs from free-range chickens, but the price of organic food means this isn't always feasible. There is a middle ground, however. If you can't eat all organic, the advice from the British Soil Association is to switch to organic versions of foods like bread and milk if these make up a large part of your diet. Also, buy organic if you're eating the foods most exposed to pesticides – squashy fruits like

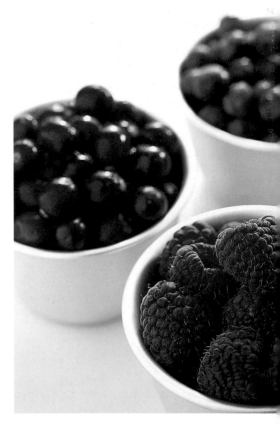

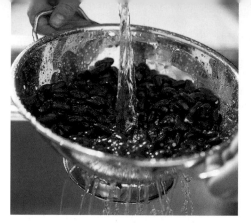

ENZYME-STIMULATING FOODS

There's more to healthy detoxing than just eating foods that are low in toxins. By choosing particular kinds of food, you can dramatically enhance the efficiency of your natural detox system. As explained earlier, much of the processing of toxins in our body occurs in the liver, where enzymes transform them into water-soluble forms that can be readily excreted. Eating particular foods can boost the levels of these enzymes that you produce. What's more, many enzyme-stimulating foods further enhance detox by actually binding with the toxins and carrying them out of the body. Combine this with the foods that stimulate your bowel and kidneys to work more efficiently, and those that neutralize harmful free radicals, and you've got the equivalent of a toxin vacuum-cleaner working hard to improve your health.

strawberries or blackberries, which absorb them more readily, and salad crops, which are heavily treated to prevent crop destruction. In the USA, the Food and Drug Administration has also ranked bell peppers, spinach, cherries, apples and peaches as often showing higher than normal pesticide residues, so you may want to switch to organic versions of these too.

For other fruits and vegetables, simply cleaning them well can help reduce pesticide residue. To do this, wash them under running water and use a small produce brush (or a new nail brush) to scrub the skins. Also, be careful where you buy fruit and vegetables – produce from roadside stalls, or shops on busy roads that display wares outside, can actually be polluted by heavy metals from car exhaust fumes. Finally, as we've met in humans, toxins in animals are also stored in fat. Therefore you should aim to eat only lean cuts of meat and also try to cut off any noticeable bits of fat. Do all of the above – or even just half of it – and you'll start to substantially lower your body's toxic load.

CHOOSING DETOX FOODS

Which foods carry out these roles? Well, practically every fruit and vegetable fights toxins in some way, but some positively excel at it. The lists on pages 17–19 will introduce you to the ultimate toxin-fighting foods. If you're not following one of our specialist detox plans at any point, incorporating four or five portions of these foods in your diet every day will still help to keep your system working at full strength and reduce the toxic load your body is under. If you are following a detox plan, you'll see how these and other detox foods can dramatically boost the plan's success.

'Produce from roadside stalls, or shops on busy roads that display wares outside, can actually be polluted by the heavy metals from traffic exhaust fumes.'

Top 10 detox foods

These ten detox foods have been shown to provide the best all-round nutrients that will work hard to get rid of the toxins in your body.

1 **APPLE** Scientists in the Ukraine have used apples to purify the area around Chernobyl after the nuclear leak.
Contains **Vitamin C and quercetin**, antioxidant nutrients that lower fat and cholesterol levels.
Pectin a fibre also found in citrus fruits, beets and berries, that binds heavy metals (such as lead and mercury) in the colon and encourages their excretion. Also helps the body excrete food additives, including tartrazine, which is linked to hyperactivity, migraine and asthma in children.

2 **AVOCADO** *Contains* **Glutathione**, an antioxidant that fights free radicals. This combines with fat-soluble toxins, particularly alcohol, to make them water-soluble. Levels of glutathione decrease as we age (that's why hangovers worsen as we get older): researchers at the University of Michigan in Ann Arbor, USA, found that elderly people, whose levels of glutathione were higher, were healthier. They were also less likely to suffer from arthritis, which many experts believe is a disease aggravated by excess toxicity.

3 **ARTICHOKE** Increases bile production. One of the jobs of bile is to carry toxins to the bowel where they can be excreted; according to research, artichoke can increase bile flow by 127 per cent 30 minutes after being eaten.
Contains **Antioxidant chemicals**. Studies from the University of Tubingen in Germany show that damage to the liver caused by free radicals is dramatically lessened when artichoke extracts are present.

4 **BEETROOT** Beetroot has been used for many years by Roman civilizations as a blood-purifying tonic. Ingredients in it may also absorb toxic metals. At Leadville, a polluted mine site in Colorado, USA, beets and other crops such as carrot and banana are being used to filter 70 per cent of pollutants from water.
Contains **Methionine**, which helps to reduce cholesterol levels and purify natural waste products from the body.

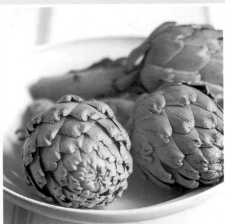

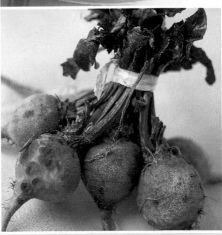

Betanin, which helps the rate at which the liver can break down fatty acids. This takes pressure off the organ, allowing it to fight more dangerous toxins.

5 CRUCIFEROUS VEGETABLES

Cabbage, kale, brussels sprouts, spinach and cauliflower are all cruciferous vegetables, and are very powerful detoxers. A study at Cornell University in the USA found that brussels sprouts inhibited aflatoxin, a toxic mould linked to liver cancer. Cruciferous vegetables have also neutralized nitrosamines in cigarette smoke. *Contains* **Glucosinolates**, which prompt the liver to produce vital enzymes.

6 GARLIC *Contains* **Allicin** is

created when garlic is crushed, and it converts into a sulphur-based compound when it enters the body. Toxins such as mercury, certain food additives and chemical versions of the hormone oestrogen bind with sulphur, enabling the body to excrete the whole package. Sulphur also helps keep the body alkaline, which can help fight cravings caused by nicotine addiction.

7 KIWI FRUIT *Contains* **Vitamin C**, a powerful antioxidant, which

also helps the body manufacture the vital detoxer glutathione (see Avocado, page 17). A study published in the *American Journal of Nutrition* found that when people were given 500mg of vitamin C a day levels of glutathione increased by 50 per cent in just two weeks.

8 PRUNES These are the ultimate antioxidant food and provide twice as

many antioxidants as blueberries, their nearest competitor.
Contains: **Tartaric acid**, a natural laxative. **Dihydropheyl isatin**, which triggers the intestine to contract. This and tartaric acid combined reduce the time faeces stays in the system, thereby reducing the risk of toxic reabsorption.

9 SEAWEED Studies at McGill University in Montreal, Canada, have

shown that seaweeds will bind in the body with radioactive waste. These wastes can reach us via food that has been grown where water or soil has been contaminated. *Contains*: **Minerals** in high doses, such as **iron, iodine, calcium** and **magnesium. Alginates**: if your body doesn't get minerals from your diet, it will try to extract them from any heavy metals it takes in. Fortunately seaweed alginates have been shown to bind with heavy metals, which facilitates their excretion.

10 WATERCRESS Watercress increases detox enzymes in the body,

and may act directly on particular toxins. When smokers were given 170g (6oz) of watercress a day at the Norwich Food Research Centre in the UK, they excreted higher than average levels of known carcinogens in their urine.
Contains: **Chlorophyll**, which helps build healthy red blood cells, boosting circulation.

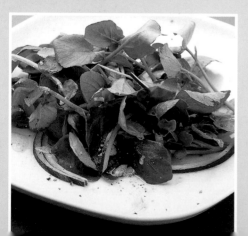

Alfalfa. High in a fibre called plantix, alfalfa has the ability to bind to toxins including some drugs and food additives. This isn't the only benefit, as it is also rich in the minerals, amino acids and fatty acids our body needs for good health and detoxing.

Asparagus. Rich in vitamin C, asparagus is also packed with fibre and the antioxidant rutin, as well as being another rich source of glutathione. Research at the Vegetable Research Unit at Cornell University, USA, shows that it stimulates the kidneys and bowel, increasing the rate at which toxins leave the body.

Bananas. Exceptionally high in minerals, bananas can reduce the uptake of heavy metals. Bananas also provide potassium, which helps to regulate fluid in the body and reduce fluid retention. The less fluid you retain the more toxins you excrete.

Bran cereals. A bowl of bran cereal contains 15g (½oz) of fibre – half the recommended daily amount. This is great for detox, because fibre cleans the bowel and stimulates its movements, decreasing the time food spends there and so reducing the risk of toxin reabsorption. Wholegrain cereals have also been proven to contain high levels of antioxidants.

Brazil nuts. The antioxidant nutrient selenium is a vital detox nutrient because it neutralizes free radicals created in the body,

WATER

We need water to flush toxins through our system, yet most of us spend the day dehydrated. You've probably heard that eight glasses of water a day is the required amount, but just aim to drink a glass of something as often as you can. Remember that it's not just plain water that hydrates us – milk is 84 per cent water, decaffeinated cola is 99 per cent water and herbal teas are 99 per cent water. They all work. You can also eat high-water foods like watermelon, celery, cucumber, pears and grapes to boost your water supply and also provide vitamins.

particularly those caused by smoking. We used to get selenium in our diet from vegetables, but levels in soil are now low. Brazil nuts are therefore the best source. Just two contain the 50mg we need daily.

Carrots. Vital sources of the antioxidants alpha- and beta-carotene, carrots also seem to be able to mop up heavy metals in the body. They also reduce cholesterol levels in the blood, which, in turn, lowers the risk of arterial furring and promotes heart health.

Eggs. These are important because they contain high levels of a substance called lecithin, which helps improve fat digestion in the body (this aids the liver) and also improves liver function. Eggs also include a detoxifier called cysteine, which is particularly potent against alcohol.

Tofu. As well as being a healthy low-fat source of protein, tofu seems to have the ability to bind to heavy metals. Research from the Harvard School of Public Health in the USA found lead levels were 11 per cent less in the bodies of people who ate 700g (1½lb) of tofu a week.

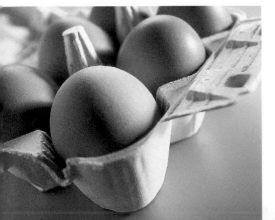

exercise and detox

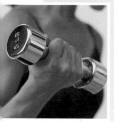

Most of us think of exercise as a way to strengthen our muscles and lose weight or body fat, but it can also be used as a way to strengthen our detox system and lose toxins. To explain how, it's best to split exercise into two types: aerobic exercise – that includes running, walking, swimming and sports – and Eastern exercise, particularly yoga.

AEROBIC EXERCISE

Whether it be running, gentle walking, swimming, tennis, squash or aerobics classes, traditional exercise has major health benefits in the body. It strengthens the heart and lungs, it builds bones, boosts the immune system, helps you sleep and even causes you to live longer. However, aerobic exercise also helps stimulate detox processes in the following ways.

- **It encourages sweating.** At rest, you lose 0.003 litres of sweat an hour, but during an hour's exercise, you can lose as much as a litre (2 pints). While 99 per cent of sweat is water, the other 1 per cent contains minerals and toxins. Therefore, the more you sweat the more toxins you will potentially excrete.
- **It makes you breathe faster.** As you exercise, your muscles produce toxic byproducts like carbon dioxide and lactic acid. When your body detects these, it actually stimulates the part of the brain that controls breathing to work faster to expel them. As you expel these toxins, others that are processed within your lungs can follow.
- **It stimulates the bowel.** In studies at the University of Maryland, USA, bowel transit time (the time it takes for things to pass through the system) was increased by 60

per cent. No one know exactly why this occurs, but it's good news for detoxers.

- **It causes safe breakdown of fat.** If you burn more calories than you take in, fat is released for the use of energy. The sudden breakdown of fat caused by crash diets leads to a sudden rush of toxins into the system that the body can't handle. By breaking fat down more slowly, moderate exercise helps to release toxins gradually.
- **It stimulates the lymphatic system.** Unlike the circulatory system, the lymphatic system does not have a pump that propels the lymph around the body. Instead it relies on muscle contraction to push it through the body – which occurs as you exercise.

All of the above factors, when combined, dramatically improve the functioning of your detox system. Before you start to train for a marathon, however, it's important to realize that, like everything to do with detoxing, moderation is the key. Studies have shown that when we exercise, free radicals are formed in the body. When exercise is regular and at a low or moderate intensity, the body can easily handle these free radicals, but work out too hard or for too long and you'll put even more pressure on your detox system. To get the benefits, you should therefore aim for between 30 and 90 minutes of low to moderate intensity per workout session; and aim for three to five sessions per week. If you want to exercise more than that without harm to your detox system, it's important that you fill your diet with lots of antioxidant-packed fruits and vegetables; you may also want to take a good multivitamin supplement.

EASTERN EXERCISE

If you don't want to pound the pavement, trudge on the treadmill or plough up and down the local swimming pool, it doesn't mean you can't boost your detox potential through exercise. Instead, you can use so-called Eastern exercises like yoga, t'ai chi and qi gong, which are gentle but equally effective forms of exercise. In fact, the perfect detox programme would include a mix of both types of exercise. This section concentrates purely on yoga, partly because it is the most researched Eastern exercise and partly because it's the easiest for beginners to pick up. Its advantages are listed in the box on the right.

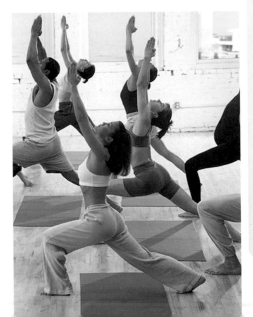

ADVANTAGES OF YOGA

- **It teaches you to breathe properly.** In a recent trial in the journal *Chest*, people with the best lung function were found to live longest. According to Dr Holger Schunemann, who conducted the trial, 'One reason for this was believed to be that the lung is a primary defence mechanism against environmental toxins. It could be that decreased pulmonary [lung] function leads to a decreased tolerance to these toxins.'
- **It stretches the muscles, releasing toxins.** Tense muscles hold toxins like lactic acid and ammonia. Stretching muscles releases these and other toxins into the bloodstream for removal. Doctors at the Bastyr's Research Institute in Seattle, USA, even prescribe yoga to patients after chemotherapy to help clear the drugs from their system.
- **It balances inner body energy.** Eastern medicine teaches that if the inner body energy – or chi – is stalled it leads to a toxic build-up that causes the body to underperform. Rebalancing the body through movement and breathing can unclog the energy and promote healthy functioning. Certain yoga postures can stimulate the detox system in this way.
- **It helps reduce stress.** A study in the *American Journal of Hypertension* found that yoga could reduce stress-induced blood pressure in less than 3 minutes. And the less stressed you are the less likely it is that you'll turn to 'comforting' toxins like alcohol or sugar.
- **It stimulates the lymphatic system.** Just like aerobic exercise, yoga involves contracting and relaxing muscles, which boosts lymph flow around the body.

Simple yoga regime

To enhance your detox programme, it's recommended that you do some form of yogic exercise. You can join an exercise class, or follow this simple 20-minute yoga regime, which is suitable for beginners. It focuses on postures that aim to cleanse the body and stimulate the detox system. For the best effects, carry out this programme at least three times a week.

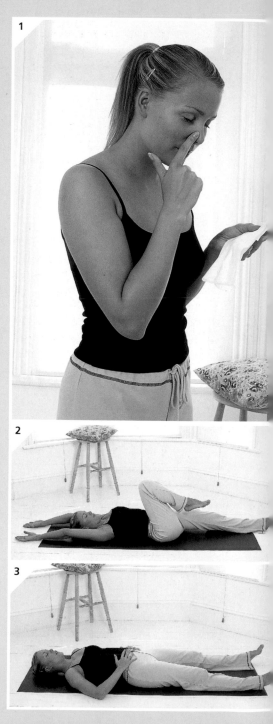

(1) ARTIFICIAL SNEEZES

Being able to breathe clearly is a vital part of yoga practice – it is seen to energize and cleanse us. This exercise decongests nasal passages and makes breathing easier.

- Take a tissue, stand up straight, then exhale deeply. Breathe in through the nose, then exhale using a series of short nasal breaths, like sneezes. Do as many as you can while exhaling.
- Inhale, then block your right nostril with your finger and exhale through the left using the 'sneeze' effect again. Inhale, block the left nostril and repeat.

(2) BASTRIKA

It's impossible to empty your lungs completely. Every time you exhale you leave at least 20 per cent 'stale' air behind – if you didn't, you'd die. However, most of us leave a lot more than 20 per cent. Instead, we exhale only 10–20 per cent. The result is that toxins in the breath spend longer in the body, and our body doesn't get all the vital oxygen it should do. This exercise helps force that old air (and toxins) out of the lungs.

- Lie on your back, legs straight. Push your chin into your neck and stretch your arms behind your head. Inhale, then quickly

22

bend your right knee up towards your chest and exhale forcefully through your mouth. Lower your knee and repeat on the left side. Finally, repeat with both knees together.

3 **YOGA BREATHING** Now you've cleansed the lungs, it's important to teach you the correct way to fill them with new air. Practise this on its own too, whenever you can.

- Lie down with your legs straight, and press your lower back into the floor. If you find this hard, bend your knees instead. Put your fingers on your navel.
- Breathe in and out a few times. Next time when you inhale aim to fill your lungs from the bottom so your tummy balloons out, then fill the middle of the lungs and finally the chest. Breathe in for a count of 5.
- Now exhale for a count of 10, letting the air out of the belly first, then the middle and finally the top of the lungs. Repeat 5 times.

4 **LEG VIBRATIONS** The heart always finds it easier to pump blood 'downhill'; the same goes for the flow of lymph, which is why toxins collect so readily in our hips, thighs, knees (in the form of arthritis) and feet (as gout). This exercise helps stimulate the blood flow in the legs.

- Lie on your back and put your legs in the air. Open them to hip-width apart and very slowly rotate your ankles to the left 5 times. Then repeat to the right.
- Now stretch your toes to the ceiling and hold them there for a count of 5. Bend your feet halfway back to their normal position and hold for 5. Now, flex your feet towards your shins and hold for 5.
- Put your feet back into their natural position, then tense your legs and try to find a point at which they naturally start to vibrate. This sounds really strange, but it will happen. The gentle vibration boosts blood flow to the groin markedly. Let yourself 'wobble' for up to 2 minutes.

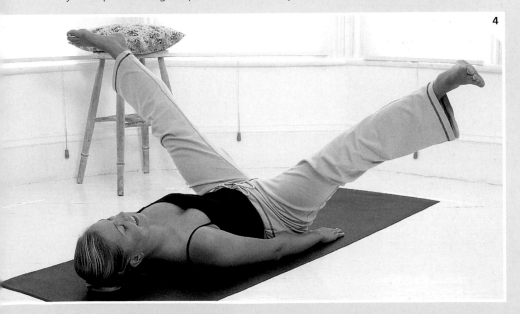

4

5A

5B

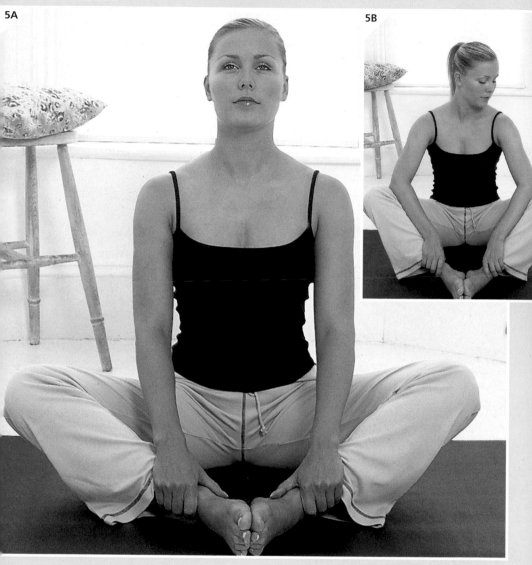

5 **BUTTERFLY** This yogic posture stimulates the blood flow around the hips and pelvic area. It both moves on the toxins that have already been released and triggers the collection of those stored around the groin. This pose also stimulates one of the major lymph-producing areas.

- **A** Sit on the floor with legs apart but knees bent and the soles of your feet together, back straight. Rest your hands on your ankles, arms by your sides.
- **B** Exhale and, as you do this, bring your knees upwards so they press against your arms. Inhale and press them back down. Do this 10 times.

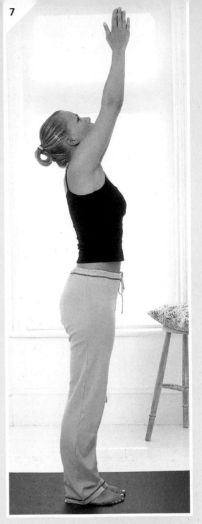

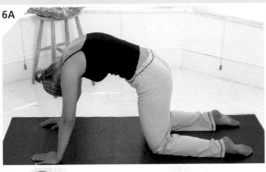

6A

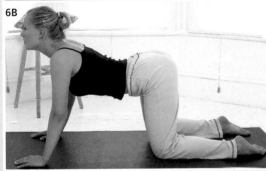

6B

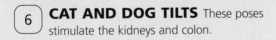

6 **CAT AND DOG TILTS** These poses stimulate the kidneys and colon.

- **A** Kneel on all fours. Keep your elbows locked and your neck straight. Exhale and, as you do this, round your upper back so that your head drops downwards between your hands. Keep your tummy and buttocks tight.
- **B** Now inhale and, as you do, push your body down and up to gently arch your back and straighten your arms. Lead with your chin as you do this. It's as if you're trying to dip under a rope. Do the whole sequence 4 times.

7 **SKYTOWER** This releases toxins down the arms and throughout the upper body.

- Stand up straight with your feet together and arms by your sides, palms facing out. Raise your arms to shoulder height, then above your head. Push your palms together, pointing your fingers skywards and stretch up through your body. Hold for 5 seconds. Exhale and repeat 5 times.

8 FISHHOOK

This stimulates the blood and lymph flow in the armpit, another major point of elimination for the body.

- **A** Stand with your legs wide apart and your feet pointing straight ahead. Breathe in, stretch out your arms and bring them up to shoulder height. Exhale and, as you do this, drop your left arm to your side.
- **B** Inhale and lift your right arm up alongside your head (close to your ear), twisting it so your palm faces the sky. Keep your hips facing forward and bend gently sideways. Hold for 5–10 seconds, exhale, then return to the starting point. Repeat on the other side.

9 COBRA

This exercise is the ultimate detox move and aims to move any unprocessed toxins to the kidneys, liver and bowel.

- **A** Lie on your front, head on the floor, hands under your shoulders. Your heels are together and your buttocks clenched.
- **B** Exhale and roll your head gently off the floor. Inhale and lift your head, shoulders and your chest off the floor by extending your arms and gently arching your back. Exhale and lower yourself back down.
- **C** When you reach your starting position, gently push backwards and sit on your heels, so you feel a stretch along your back. Relax in this pose for a few seconds.
- **D** Repeat step **C** 3 times. The last time, relax for a little longer and then slowly rise up on to your feet, and 'unfold' your body to standing. Your head should remain bowed as you do this and be brought up slowly only when you are upright. Spend 1 minute carrying out yoga breathing (see page 23) and you're done.

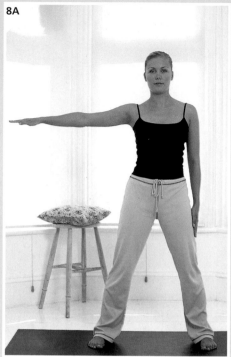

8A

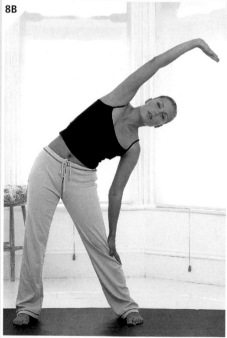

8B

9A

9B

9C

9D

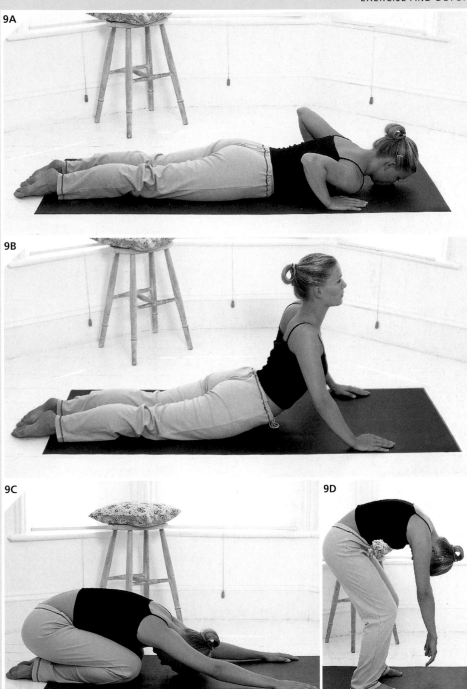

external detoxing

Detoxing your body is not just about what goes on with your body internally. Although stimulating the detox process through diet, exercise and nutrition is the most important part of the process, what happens to the body externally can also play a part. Body-brushing, heat treatments and massage are three excellent ways that you can use to stimulate detox from the outside.

BODY-BRUSHING AND BODY SCRUBS

Every day an estimated 450g (1lb) of toxins leave the body in sweat carried out through the skin – but only if the pores, through which sweat travels, are clear. Every day our skin cells regenerate; old ones die, and new ones are created, pushing the old cells away. However, as we age the process slows down. Skin cells die, but new ones to replace them don't appear as rapidly. This means that the cells aren't pushed off the surface, so it's harder for them to shed, and they build up. Cosmetically this creates a dull appearance, but in terms of detox it can cause a blockage that reduces the amount of toxins excreted from the cells. Removing dead skin cells is therefore an important part of the detox process.

1 Body scrubs. In health spas, it's common for a little damp sea salt to be used on dry skin (and not on wet skin as most people think). This is then rinsed off in a shower to reveal smooth and revitalized skin.

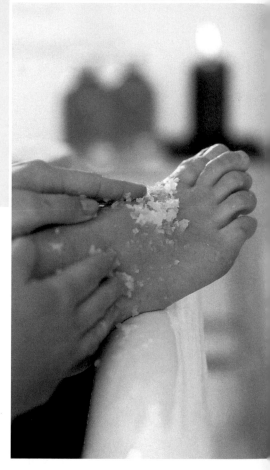

2 Body-brushing. Choose a natural-bristled brush with medium-hard bristles. Synthetic bristles or those that are too hard can scratch the skin. While the skin is dry, use long, firm (but not hard) strokes to brush the whole body one area at a time. Always start with the soles of your feet, because stimulating these actually starts the lymph flowing. Brush smoothly 4–5 times, always in the direction of the heart, moving around the whole body part. Do this around your calves, then your thighs and hips. Now do your arms, chest, torso and back. Finally, brush your stomach. Once you've finished, shower or at least rinse the skin off. As well as obviously cleaning the skin, the repeated motion of brushing or scrubbing the body causes the speed of the circulation to increase (helping flush toxins out of the system faster), and this is also believed to promote lymph flow.

HEAT TREATMENTS

Sauna and steam treatments are used in countries like Sweden and Finland to help keep the body healthy and toxin-free. There are certainly some research studies that say they can make a difference: during a sauna the heart output increases by up to 75 per cent, boosting blood flow, and 70 per cent of that blood reaches the skin. Any toxins carried in the blood are therefore closer to the surface of the body and, so the theory goes, will be more likely to be sweated out.

So how should you use saunas and steams? While intensive detox regimes claim that saunas of two to three hours can also break down fat stores and help release pesticides and heavy metals into the system, such a long length of time is not recommended by this book. Not only have we already seen that releasing large doses of chemicals into the system confuses the body, but sitting for that long in a sauna without medical supervision could be harmful. If you want to use saunas to help your detox process, stick to 10–20 minutes at a time at a heat you can bear. Don't eat a heavy meal or drink alcohol before the treatment, but do drink plenty of water before, during and after your session. You can lose 30ml (1floz) of water or more in a sauna, which is enough to dehydrate the

SMOKERS AND SAUNAS

When smokers leave a sauna they often leave a yellow tar residue on the towels. And when Finlandia Sauna replace the benches in their public saunas they often find a fine layer of black tar underneath. If that doesn't make you want to stop smoking, nothing will.

body and start to slow urine production, which defeats the object. Finally, if you have any medical problems that involve your heart, blood pressure, respiratory system or skin, see your doctor before using saunas or steams to check if they are safe for you. Saunas and steam rooms are not recommended for pregnant women.

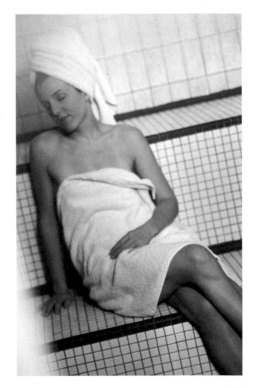

MASSAGE

When it comes to detox, massage works on two main levels. First, massage helps reduce stress, so it can be used to reduce cravings for the toxin-filled goodies such as alcohol, cigarettes or sugar that many of us turn to when we're under pressure. Second, the pressure of the hands on the body can act in the same way as exercise or body-brushing to stimulate blood circulation and lymph flow. Chinese research has also shown that, when the body is massaged, the temperature of the skin increases, and this widens the gaps between the cells of the body. These gaps are where the lymph flows, and by increasing their size you stimulate the flow of lymph, allowing it to feed more nutrients to the cells and collect more waste products from the area.

So how do you use massage to help you detox? The most important thing to do is to choose the right type. Massage comes in many different forms, and while something like a sport massage will help

relieve the pain of an injury, it won't have maximum benefit for detoxing.

Manual lymph drainage. This is the most beneficial type of massage for detoxing. It uses a mixture of long gentle strokes with pulsing techniques to focus completely on stimulating the flow of lymph. Full manual lymph drainage must be carried out by a specialist, or the lymph can be damaged, so ask at your nearest natural health store or centre for recommendations or check your local telephone directory for practitioners. However, you can carry out a very gentle form of lymph massage yourself (see the fluid-busting massage on pages 32–33).

Aromatherapy massages. These treatments apply pressure to the body to increase blood flow while scented oils with various detox properties are absorbed into the skin (see pages 36–37).

Although you'll get the best results from massage if you go to a professional, there are some basic techniques that can be learned at home. The simple neck and shoulder massage that is shown opposite can be carried out on yourself if you need to de-stress or detox from something like a hangover. Then, there's a fuller back massage regime that you can carry out on someone else – or, more importantly, that you can teach someone to perform on you when you need to relax or want to deliver the healing power of aromatherapy oils to a wider area of your body.

'Manual lymph drainage is the most beneficial type of massage for detoxing.'

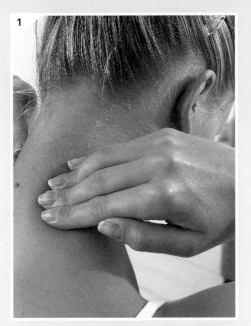

Simple do-it-yourself neck and shoulder massage

You don't need any oil to carry out this massage, but if you want to use one, try the de-stressing blend (see page 70) or add the ingredients from the energizing bath blend (see page 95) to 12ml (½floz) of carrier oil.

1 Tilt your head back and, with the palms and fingers of each hand, gently squeeze each side where your neck meets your shoulders. Still squeezing, gently tilt your head forwards. Hold for a few seconds, then tilt your head back up.

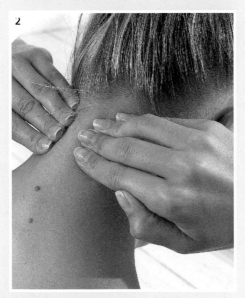

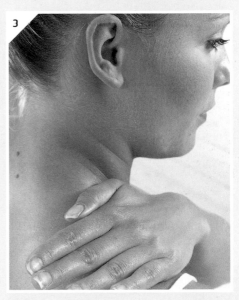

2 Stroke the back of your neck for 30 seconds. Then use the fingers of both your hands to make deep circular pressures all around the neck area, steering clear of the spine itself.

3 Place your left hand on your right shoulder and squeeze the muscle. Release, then tap the area 4–5 times with the palm of your hand. Repeat the process on the other side.

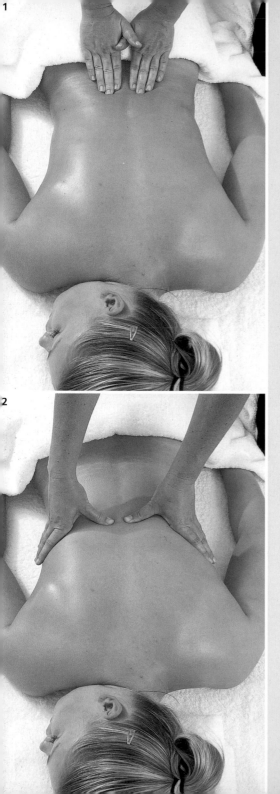

Back massage

Before you start, make sure the room is warm, and dim the lights to aid relaxation. The person to be massaged – your massage partner – should lie on their front, on a firm but supportive surface. Cover their lower body with towels to keep them warm. The masseur should use a massage oil to help their hands move smoothly across the skin. Either use a specialist detox blend or make your own (see page 35).

1 Make contact with the skin. Ensuring that your hands are warm, place them very gently on your partner's back at the base of the spine. Leave them there for a few seconds. Now, with your fingers together and the whole of the hand touching the back, make one constant movement to slide your hands up the spine. Sweep around the shoulder blades and back down the spine. Do this 10 times.

2 Place your thumbs either side of your partner's spine. Move them up 7.5cm (3in) and gently rotate each thumb. Continue up the spine like this until you reach the top. Bring your hands back to the starting position by sweeping them down the sides of the back, then repeat the thumb move. Do this 5 times.

Warning It is essential that whoever is performing the massage does not press on the spine itself, but only on the muscles that are on either side of the spine.

3

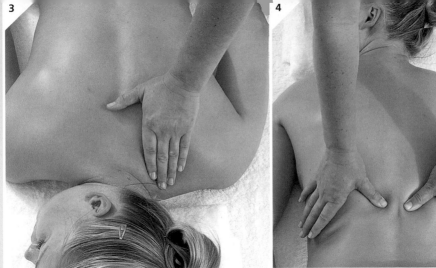

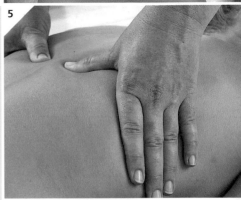

3 Sweep your hands up to your partner's shoulder blades. Then, working on one shoulder at a time, push the heel of your hand against their shoulder blade, pushing up to the top of the shoulder.

4 Now, without breaking contact with your partner's back, move so you are standing in front of their head. Depending on the difference in your height, you may have to 'walk' your fingers up their body to retain contact while you do this. Now, starting with your hands at the top of your partner's back, push them very gently down the spine, around the small of the back, then up the sides of the body. Do this 10 times.

5 Bring your hands back to the top of the spine and place your thumbs at the top. In one movement push your thumbs down the spine, pressing fairly hard on the muscles (but not so it hurts). When you reach the base of the spine, bring your hands back up by sliding them around the sides of the body. Do this 5 times.

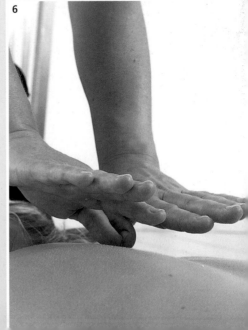

6 Finish by repeating the sliding movement in step 4 10 times. Break contact with your partner gently, one finger at time, then cover them with a warm towel and leave them to relax.

using aromatherapy

The sense of smell is very important to the healthy functioning of the body. It has been shown that scents improve energy, clarify thinking, increase libido and invoke memories that can change our moods. Any of the estimated 400,000 scents we can be exposed to can provoke these reactions, but the most potent actions seem to come from the essential oils used in aromatherapy.

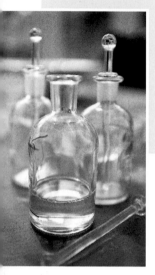

The idea behind aromatherapy is that substances within essential oils can physically stimulate actions in the brain or body, so by choosing the right oil you can cause the body to act in a particular way. It sounds strange, but it has been proven in a number of scientific studies. For example, burns treated with lavender oil have been shown to heal faster than normal. When sedative essential oils are used in hospitals, patients fall asleep faster and stay asleep for longer than usual. When exercisers sniff peppermint oil before they work out, they exercise harder, and find it easier. In terms of detox, essential oils have been used for years to deal with toxic symptoms. Advisors to the Roman emperors used the oil of black pepper to help their charges deal with over-indulgence, while early Greek doctors used juniper as a diuretic.

It's clear to see from the above that aromatherapy oils can play a part in keeping us healthy and detoxed, so how can you use their powers? Here are the three most commonly used methods.

INHALATIONS

These are great for their mental effects, or if you're suffering from a problem like a hangover. Add 8–10 drops of neat oil to a bowl of hot water and place your face over the water (at least 10cm/4in from the surface) and breathe slowly and deeply for 5–10 minutes. For a simple pick-up, you can also add a few drops to a tissue and inhale.

MASSAGE

You can massage all over the body, or, if you want to have a particular effect on a particular organ (the liver or the kidneys, for example), you should focus your massage on the area in which it's located. Remember, however, that very few essential oils can be used neat on the skin. Most cause irritation if you do this, and some can even be toxic. Instead, mix them with a 'carrier oil' first.

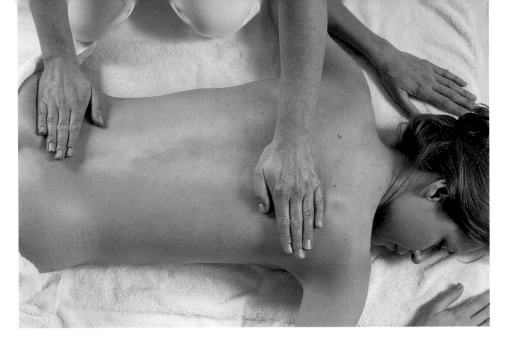

Carrier oils are oils with no healing powers; they just carry the essential oil safely onto the skin. Good carrier oils include grapeseed, sweet almond or wheatgerm, and you should use half the number of drops of essential oil as there are millilitres of carrier oil. So, if you have a 25ml bottle of carrier oil, you would add 12–13 drops of your chosen oil (or, if you are making a blend of oils, 12–13 drops in total). It's important to do a skin-patch test before using any oil to check that you're not sensitive to it. Dab a little behind your ear and wait 24 hours to check that no itching or rash has developed.

BATHING

This is the simplest way to use aromatherapy. For maximum benefit run your bath, sprinkle three to six drops of essential oil on the surface and then agitate the water to ensure that you don't get a concentrated dose of the oil on your skin. Bathing can be used to treat many problems because the oils are absorbed by the skin, and the heat of the water releases the scent – this will help with problems like stress, low energy or hangovers.

Warning Some aromatherapy oils can interfere with medical conditions, including epilepsy and diabetes. If you have a medical condition, seek advice from a registered aromatherapist before treating yourself. Many oils are also not suitable if you're pregnant. Again, if you are not 100 per cent certain that the oil you want to use is safe, seek professional advice. Finally, essential oils should never be taken internally.

'Aromatherapy oils can play a part in keeping us healthy and detoxed.'

Top 10 detox oils

These are the oils that can play a role in detoxing. You can use them on their own or make up blends, either by using the tips about which oils they work well with or by following the specific blends given in some of the detox plans (see pages 42–125).

1 ANGELICA

Invigorating for the lymphatic system, angelica is particularly good at getting rid of toxins after illness. It will also act on fluid retention and stimulate the skin to sweat. It's also believed to be a tonic for the liver and spleen. You'll like it if you like sweet, musky smells, but don't use it if you are pregnant or going out into the sun, since it makes the skin photosensitive.

Blends well with: grapefruit, lemon and mandarin oils.

2 BLACK PEPPER

If your colon is acting up, black pepper oil may help strengthen things. It's used to restore tone to the colon muscles and encourages bowel movements. The ancient Romans used it to help people overcome food poisoning, and to help them digest heavy meals and red meat. It is also a good stimulant for the circulation. Don't use black pepper oil neat on the skin as it can irritate. If you're using it in massage or bath blends, add only one or two drops and always mix it well in a carrier oil.

Blends well with: cypress, grapefruit and lemon.

3 CYPRESS

With its pine-needle scent, this oil's job is to regulate the overall fluid balance of the body. This means that it is excellent at tackling water retention and allergy symptoms like runny noses. The good thing about this is that, although it has diuretic properties, it doesn't dehydrate the body. It also helps to strengthen the circulation and liver. This oil is not recommended for use during any stage of pregnancy.

Blends well with: juniper, lemon and orange.

4 FENNEL

A big toxin-buster, fennel has been traditionally used to detox the poisons from insect or snake bites, but for most of us its power lies in its ability to cleanse the body after you have eaten or drunk too much. Hangovers can be helped by a massage blend including fennel. Use it sparingly, however, since in high doses it can be quite toxic and, if you have sensitive skin, it can irritate. It shouldn't be used in pregnancy or by anyone with epilepsy.

Blends well with: lemon and juniper.

5 GERANIUM

Strongly floral, this scent detoxes the body from within. It's a good diuretic (helping you to pass water) and helps stimulate both the liver and the kidneys;

it's an immune-booster, stimulating the lymphatic system; and it also thins the blood, making the blood easier to pump around the body. Geranium also balances the body mentally; research carried out in Japan has shown that when used on people who were stressed it calmed the body, but when used on those who needed stimulating it did just that.

Blends well with: angelica, grapefruit and orange.

6 GRAPEFRUIT

An energizing and reviving oil, grapefruit is a lymph stimulant. It also helps to control water levels in the body, and can reduce fluid retention and increase urine flow. Furthermore, it's believed to stimulate bile production in the liver, and has been used to help withdrawal symptoms in detox clinics. However, if you're using it to help fight weight gain caused by fluid, be careful – its citrus scent can be an appetite stimulant and actually work against you. It also makes skin sensitive to sunlight.

Blends well with: geranium.

7 JUNIPER

The liver-boosting oil, this has even been used to help boost healing after liver disease. It can help feelings of over-indulgence and hangovers and it also helps clear the intestine. It can help suppress the appetite so, if you're on a detox plan that involves cutting down on particular foods, it could help to make things easier for you. Juniper has diuretic properties and it helps to boost the kidneys. Do not use juniper during pregnancy, or over-use it generally, since its powerful diuretic action can over-tax the kidneys.

Blends well with: cypress, geranium, grapefruit and orange.

8 LEMON

An all-round body cleanser, lemon helps strengthen the liver and the kidneys, and thins the blood, boosting circulation. It also stimulates white blood cells, boosting the immune system. It fights acidity in the system (the body often becomes acidic when we eat lots of red meat), which is good news because an acidic body is more prone to creating those free radicals.

Blends well with: fennel and juniper.

9 MANDARIN

Renowned for helping combat feelings of fragility and loss of balance, mandarin can help soothe many of the symptoms of increasing toxicity. It also has its own cleansing actions; it has a stimulating effect on the liver, promotes bile production and aids in breaking down fat. If you suffer from wind, it can help the body expel gas. It is one of the few oils that is believed to be totally safe in pregnancy and can be used on children effectively – although you should cautiously stick to using just tiny amounts in both instances.

Blends well with: black pepper, grapefruit and lemon.

10 PATCHOULI

A very strong diuretic, patchouli helps the body to fight fluid retention and cellulite as well as flushing toxins through the kidneys. It's an appetite balancer, which can help reduce over-indulgence in rich foods and alcoholic drinks. It also balances the mind, giving energy when it's needed and sedating when stress levels are particularly high; as a result, it can treat symptoms and any major cause of toxic overload in the body.

Blends well with: black pepper and geranium.

using supplements

Food is your most important weapon in detoxing your body. It's the way your body expects to get everything it needs to function normally, so therefore it is the most effective way of giving it all it needs. Some herbs, vitamins and other supplements, however, can help support the food you eat when trying to detox. If you walk into a health food store, you'll see loads of these packed in pills, potions, teas and powders, and it can be very confusing. So, six of the best general supplements you can use to aid your detox programme are recommended and described in this section. This doesn't mean that you should head out to the health food store, buy them all and take every pill till you rattle. Each supplement has a different use, and some should be taken only for

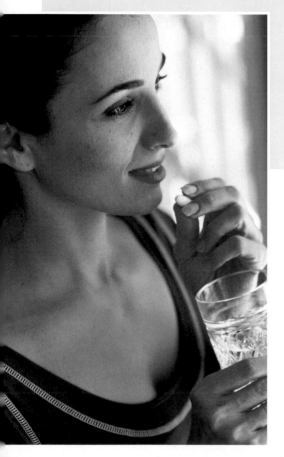

a short time if you feel you need help in a particular area. If you want to do a major detox you can combine the supplements but, normally, it's a good idea never to take more than two supplements (excluding multivitamins, which won't cause problems if taken alongside other supplements) at any one time.

CHLORELLA

Made from algae, chlorella is a high source of protein, vitamins (including antioxidants like A, C and E) and chlorophyll, which increases oxygen in the blood. However, its main detox power comes from its ability to bind to particular toxins. Japanese research has shown that up to ten times more cadmium (a heavy metal usually found in soil that you take in smoke from tobacco if you smoke, or even smoke passively) is excreted when chlorella is taken. It's also been shown to act against lead, mercury and chemical pollutants, and may have similar results to watercress in helping to detox other harmful cigarette ingredients.

When to take it: the recommended dose is one to three tablets taken daily with meals, or a tablespoonful of powder mixed with drinks or added to smoothies. Like multivitamins, it can be taken every day, but it's specifically helpful if you've been exposed to smoke or need to boost energy.

DANDELION

To reduce fluid levels in the body, pills and potions are generally not recommended. The reason for this is that most diuretics also cause the body to leach vital potassium stores, which is bad for your heart. Dandelion is the exception to this: it contains high levels of potassium, so does not cause loss of the mineral. Herbalists also believe dandelion helps to increase bile production, while Japanese research has shown that it can double the amount of one detoxifying enzyme produced in the liver. It's also high in antioxidants. Dandelion tea is probably the easiest way to consume dandelion, but its peppery leaves can also be eaten in salads.

When to take it: if you feel bloated or suffer from cellulite and fluid retention. It can also be used to reduce the symptoms of pre-menstrual syndrome. Dandelion tea can

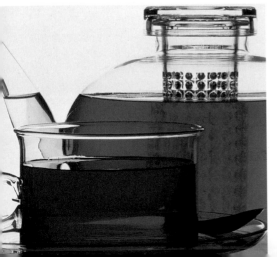

also be drunk as an overall health beverage to boost antioxidant levels.

MILK THISTLE

There are over 30 herbs that claim to help strengthen the liver, but the one that has been researched the most is milk thistle. Full of an active compound called silymarin, which is found in the seeds of the plant, milk thistle has been shown to help make the liver cells less permeable to toxins, preventing damage from occurring. It reduces destruction of glutathione, which helps increase the speed at which the body can reduce toxins – particularly alcohol and pollutants. In Germany, it's also a common treatment against cirrhosis of the liver.

When to take it: you can take it daily if you really feel you are suffering from toxin overload. A 140–200mg dose three times daily is the recommended amount. Otherwise, it's best used as a precursor for alcohol. If you know you are going to drink a lot on a particular day, take 300–600mg in the few days beforehand. If alcohol overload sneaks up on you, however, make sure you take a 600mg dose when you get home, 300mg the morning after and 300mg in the evening, which will help to eliminate it faster. If you still feel unwell the day after, repeat this dosage.

MULTIVITAMINS

Detoxing uses up massive amounts of nutrients in the body. If you smoke more than 20 cigarettes a day, 40 per cent of your daily vitamin C intake is used to try to neutralize the damage that is caused as a result. When the liver processes toxins, free radicals are formed, which destroy not only vitamin C but also vitamin A, vitamin E and the mineral selenium. Toxins also attack nutrients. Alcohol, for example, stops B

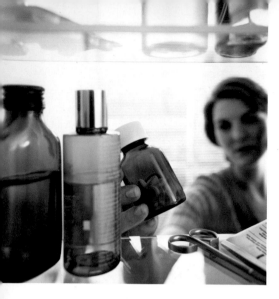

vitamins being absorbed and encourages the excretion of calcium. All of this reduces the nutrients in your body, which is bad news because studies show that people who have the highest levels of nutrients in their diet are healthiest and live longest. Therefore, taking a good multivitamin alongside your detox diet can improve your overall health and the success of your detox programme. It's also safer than taking individual pills. This is because studies have shown that taking individual nutrients can actually harm the body, as they throw it out of its natural balance.

When to take them: daily with food.

PROBIOTICS

When the body breaks down food, it turns it into tiny molecules that aren't seen as a threat. But, if a condition called 'leaky gut' occurs, this changes. In leaky gut, the intestines become permeable and large food molecules can get into the bloodstream. These then reach the liver, which sees them as a toxin and wastes energy trying to tackle them – allowing other toxins to build up. Probiotics help

tackle leaky gut by increasing levels of vital digestive bacteria in the gut; the more of these there are the less likely it is that the condition will occur.

When to take them: if you have a lot of digestive problems like stomach bloating, diarrhoea or abdominal cramps, leaky gut may play a part. It's believed that many allergy sufferers also suffer from leaky gut and may benefit from probiotics. They do not need to be taken indefinitely; instead, take them for two to three weeks, which is enough time to replenish the gut. You should also take them after a course of antibiotics. Probiotics should be taken about half an hour before you eat.

PSYLLIUM HUSKS

Used most commonly in a laxative form, psyllium husks contain high levels of soluble fibre. When they combine with water, they swell in the bowel, absorbing toxins but also stimulating the bowel to work, so the toxins are passed out more quickly. Studies have shown that when psyllium is taken, bowel transit time can be almost halved.

When to take them: if you have problems with constipation, or if you have dramatically over-indulged. It is safe to take it every day because, unlike many laxatives, psyllium does not make the bowel 'lazy' (which can cause further problems when the laxative is stopped), but it's best used only when necessary. It can also be used as a supplement to help reduce cholesterol. Take 5g twice daily, half an hour before meals, diluted in plenty of water. Psyllium may cause some allergic reactions. If you have hayfever or rhinitis, it may cause symptoms. It can also trigger asthma attacks, so is best avoided by asthmatics. Also, don't take it at the same time as probiotics, since they cancel each other out.

side-effects

All the unpleasant symptoms you normally get when you're on a detox programme probably won't appear if you follow the advice in this book. Feelings of exhaustion, irritability, bad breath and so on happen not because your body is eliminating toxins but because you're starving it. Since you're not going to do that, they are unlikely to occur. However, on some of the specialist plans you may find you experience some side-effects, which are all detailed here – along with ways to alleviate them.

HEADACHES

These may occur if you give up or reduce the amount of caffeine in your diet. If you drink tea or coffee daily, the blood vessels in the brain become constricted; take the caffeine hit away and they dilate, triggering headaches. Dab a little lavender oil on your temple or buy some tiger balm, which will relieve even the worst headache.

SKIN PROBLEMS

If you come out in a rash it may not be due to toxins leaving the skin. It's more likely to be a reaction to an aromatherapy oil or a grimy body-brush. Do a skin-patch test with each oil and soak your brush in a solution of 1 tablespoon of bleach to one cup of water, then rinse well.

INCREASED URINATION

Don't panic. Generally, the more you pee the more toxins you expel. It will be most common on the Weight-loss Plan (see page 100). In food intolerances, the body conserves water to dilute the offending food. So when you eliminate them from your diet, you may urinate more. If you urinate too often, though, it may be that you are drinking water too quickly.

STOMACH PROBLEMS

If you eat four to five detox foods (see pages 17–19) a day, you'll be taking in a lot of fibre. If you get stomach cramps, reduce the amount of fibre and build up slowly. If you get cramps while taking psyllium, lower your dose or stop. On the Decaf and Stop Smoking Plans (see pages 56 and 82), you may become constipated because caffeine and smoking stimulate the bowel.

CRAVINGS

Cravings are often psychological: when people are on diets, they start to fixate on what they can and can't eat. However, if you're not eating enough, your body will crave foods it knows gives it energy fast. Eating more regularly or adding more protein to meals can reduce cravings.

DETOX BENEFITS

You'll have more energy, your skin and hair will look healthier, you'll probably lose weight and you'll sleep better. Once your first plan is finished, you'll notice how you have re-educated your body and how good you feel. It may spur you on to try some other plans.

detoxing:
THE PLANS

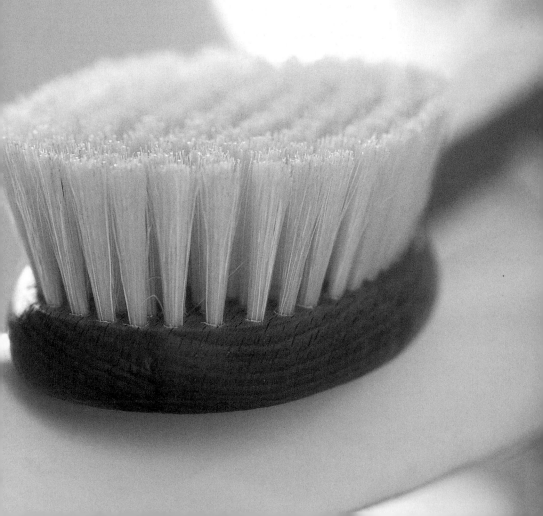

using the plans

Up until now, you've been learning the basics of detoxing, and how to integrate these into your life if you just want to boost your health generally. However, for most of us, detox means more than that. What we actually want to do when we detox is break the hold that toxins have over our body. It could be breaking the hold over the way they make us feel, the way they make us look or the way they make us behave.

That's where this part of the book comes in: it gives 14 specific plans that will help you tackle some of the major toxin problems that we all encounter in life. How they do this varies. If, for example, you're trying to beat toxic symptoms like low energy, cellulite or just feeling generally under the weather, it will give advice on how to do just that.

Which plans you choose depends on where you are in your life. If you're a party person, you'll probably focus on the alcohol-related plans – or the general cleanse you'll get from the Lighten-up Plan (see page 44). Stressed-out workers will probably turn to the Energizing Plan (see page 90) or the Stress-busting Plan (see page 66). Those of you with children may want to focus on the wider picture, looking first at how to reduce the amount of harmful pollutants you and your family are exposed to by consulting the Anti-pollution Plan (see page 48). Whichever plan you choose to try first, it will help you to take control of your life. You can then look at other areas and combine their effects to detox your body completely.

HOW THE PLANS WORK

Like the first part of the book, the plans focus on diet, nutrition and alternative therapies that will help reduce the effects

'Whichever plan you choose to try first, it will help you to take control of your life.'

of toxins. They vary in length – some take over a month, some a week, some just a day – but they will all give results. You need no specialist knowledge or equipment, just a willingness to give things a try. Some of the plans have times of the day in them; these are just to give you a structure. Each plan contains three common elements:

About... This section describes when and why you are likely to need the plan, explaining what it is trying to achieve, why it's important and why it works. Don't skip this bit – understanding what something does to your body makes it easier to see why you need to tackle it, and this will motivate you if things get tough.

The solution. This provides all the practical advice to show you how the plan can be used to best effect.

Living the detox life. Finally, in each plan there are tips on how to continue the good work after you've come off it.

lighten-up plan

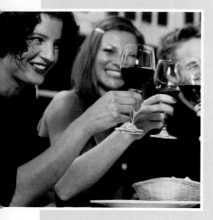

This is the detox plan for those post-Christmas feelings, for after your summer holiday, your best friend's hen or stag night or the week of your birthday – basically all those times when you've really overdone it, when you get to the point where, if you see another chocolate, you'll explode; or the smell of cooking sherry almost brings on a hangover. The Lighten-up Plan will change those feelings. It's also a good way to start the detoxing process off, and can be used for three days before any of the other plans in order to enhance their effects.

About lightening up

This plan works by bringing into play all the detox-stimulating techniques discussed in the first part of this book.

It uses diet and supplements to strengthen the liver, helping it process the toxin overload that is making you feel bad, and uses techniques like body-brushing and exercise to add to their effects. It floods the body with nutrients that you've been lacking while you've been over-indulging, and, by taking out many of the typically 'toxic' foods, it breaks bad eating behaviour before it becomes a habit. It also helps repair the digestive system, so that when you come off the plan your body will be better able to cope next time it gets attacked by alcohol, sugar or four three-course meals on the trot.

Admittedly, it's a strict programme. It's the only plan in the book where there is no red meat, no sugary foods, no wheat, no

dairy products and (ideally) no caffeine; however, at this point this is exactly what your body needs to help it recover from the last few days or weeks. Even so, it's not an unbearable plan. You are not surviving on just juices. Instead, you'll be eating five times a day with meals designed to balance your energy, so any cravings for sugar and caffeine are lessened – and if any do crop up there is advice on how to tackle them.

The solution

The daily aim of this one-week programme is to stimulate your detox system as much as possible.

Many of the things you'll do will need to be done every day; and, as this makes it slightly repetitive, a day-to-day plan has not been given. Instead, advice on what you should be doing or eating at a particular point each day is provided; if this varies, it will be made clear. It's easy once you get started.

Lighten-up programme

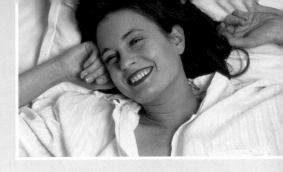

7am Wake up. Don't jump out of bed and get dressed. Your body regenerates overnight, creating natural waste products that, if released suddenly by you charging around because you're late, can tax your liver. By stretching the muscles first thing in the morning, you start the toxins moving more gently through the system. So try the following stretching programme in bed:

- Start with your feet, tensing and extending each muscle in them and then letting them relax. Now move up to your calves, again tensing and relaxing. Do the same with your thighs, buttocks, stomach. Now start with your upper body: clench then relax your hands and lower arms, then tense and relax your upper arms, and finally your shoulders. Don't clench the muscles in your neck because they are generally tense enough, but turn your head gently to the left then to the right, and repeat the other way. Clench and relax your shoulders again, your chest and your back. Shake out your muscles and get up.

7.30am Take the following supplements with a large glass of water (the first of eight glasses you'll drink over the day – try for one every hour):
- 1 multivitamin
- 1 probiotic supplement
- 140ml milk thistle (take with each meal)
These supplements start to strengthen your liver and digestive system. Leave half an hour before eating.

7.35am Have a detox bath. While bedtime may more commonly be bathtime for you, you can't have a detox bath before bed since the diuretic properties of many of the oils will keep you up all night. The good news is that the oils used in detoxing are usually energizing so, as long as the water isn't too hot, you won't feel sleepy when you're finished. Start by body-brushing while the bath runs. When it's full, add three to six drops of any of the oils listed on pages 36–37, or try a stimulating detox blend of two drops geranium oil, two drops mandarin oil and one drop grapefruit oil. Agitate the water to prevent a concentrated dose settling in any one place, then relax for 10 15 minutes.

8am Eating breakfast is vital for detoxing. Not only is it the first chance in your day to replenish all the nutrients your body used in repairing itself during the night, but it also stimulates the elimination system to start removing the debris created. A good detox breakfast contains high levels of nutrients and fibre like the three below. Choose one of these each day, but don't accompany them with tea or coffee. If you want a hot drink, try ginger or peppermint tea or chicory, all of which stimulate the body but don't contain caffeine.

- **Fibre provider.** A bowl of bran cereal with soya milk, topped with a chopped banana and some prunes.
- **Fruit salad.** Chop an apple, a slice of watermelon, a banana, a handful of grapes and a pear and mix with half a cup of unsweetened orange juice.

• **Supersmoothie.** Many detox diets use juice drinks to cleanse the system because they are easy for the body to digest, but since they include no fibre they are not nutritious enough to use as meals. Instead, if you want to drink a meal, choose a smoothie, which retains fibre. Combine a large slice of watermelon, a banana, a handful of strawberries and a glass of orange juice (you could also add a scoop of chlorella powder) in a blender and whisk until liquid.

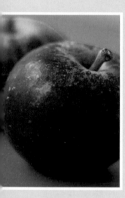

10am Snack on two pieces of fruit. Choose any fruits that you particularly like, but good detoxers include oranges, kiwi, strawberries, blueberries and apples. By eating small, regular meals and snacks, you boost the amount of nutrients you take in and also prevent sudden drops in your blood-sugar levels, which can lead to low energy and cause cravings for coffee and tea. However, if you are craving either, try a little acupressure. A good one for caffeine withdrawal is a point called 'Bigger Rushing'. You'll find this on your foot, in the valley between the big toe and the second toe. Rub it gently for a minute. If this doesn't work and you're desperate, then have a coffee; one or two cups in a day really won't hurt you.

1pm Use lunch to strengthen your detox system and also give you the energy to face the afternoon ahead. The mistake many of us make with lunch is to pack it full of carbohydrates (like bread or jacket potatoes). These are healthy choices, but too many carbohydrates in one go can make you sleepy, aggravating the natural energy dip we get mid-afternoon and causing cravings for toxin-filled foods like chocolate or biscuits. Instead, focus your lunch on detoxing fruits and vegetables, and then add a 75g (3oz) serving of low-fat protein. Start your meal with a cup or glass of either the Winter Warmer Soup or the Cleansing Juice (see box below).

Now choose one of these four bases; use as much of each vegetable as you like:
Detox Salad. Watercress, celery, cucumber, cherry tomato, artichoke hearts.
Cleansing Coleslaw. White cabbage, onion, grated carrot, sliced beetroot.
Roast energy Grill or oven-bake slices of red pepper, yellow pepper, aubergine, onion, mushrooms, until soft.
Steamed and Simple Steamed carrot, mangetout, cauliflower, spinach, asparagus.

Winter Warmer Soup
(serves one)
250ml (8floz) chicken or vegetable stock • ½ 400g (13oz) can of tomatoes • 1 carrot, sliced • ½ onion, chopped • 75g (3oz) potato, cubed • 50g (2oz) pumpkin, skinned and cubed • salt and pepper to taste
Put all the ingredients in a large pan and bring the mixture to the boil. Cover, then simmer for 20–30 minutes. Pour the mixture into a blender or food processor and blend until completely smooth. Finally, add salt and pepper to taste before serving.

Cleansing Juice
5 carrots • 1 apple • 2 stalks of celery • ½ beetroot
Juice all the ingredients until smooth, and then serve.

To whichever base you have chosen, add a 75g (3oz) portion of one the following: prawns, tuna, mussels, salmon, sardines, poached white fish, chicken, turkey, tofu, beans, lentils or one boiled or poached egg.

4pm Have another fruit snack to keep your energy up. If you normally have a sugary snack about now, you could be craving chocolate. If so, get some vanilla essence and keep it handy to sniff when a craving hits. Studies at St George's Hospital in London have shown this can help reduce the severity of chocolate cravings.

5–7pm Do some exercise. The early evening is the best time of the day for exercise, since muscles are at their warmest. Three days a week, do 30 minutes of exercise, such as swimming, running, aerobics or brisk walking. Three other days, practise some yoga (see pages 22–27). On the other day have a rest. Leave at least half an hour after exercise before eating.

7pm Use the power of carbohydrates to help you sleep, evening is the best time to eat them, so this time add a serving of carbohydrate foods (or starchy vegetables) to those detoxing fruit and vegetables.
• Choose a starter – Winter Warmer Soup or Cleansing Juice.
• Choose one of the Lunch vegetable bases.
• Add a 75g (3oz) serving of one (or a mix) of the following: brown rice, jacket potato, new potatoes, mashed potatoes, wheat-free pasta, mashed swede, roast parsnips, corn on the cob, sweetcorn, rye bread or pumpernickel bread.

9pm Take a relaxing bath. Use a little essential oil of lavender to promote both deep sleep and regeneration in your body.

Living the detox life

When it comes to the Lighten-up Plan, you probably know what it takes to live the detox life – don't drink like a fish or eat everything in sight for more than one day at a time! However, for more constructive advice, re-visit the first section of this book.

• Food toxins aren't bad for your body in small doses. Whenever possible, try to stick to 'safe' limits (see pages 8–10).
• Building four to five detox foods (see pages 17–19) into your daily diet will help strengthen your detox system ready for any over-indulgences. You are then less likely to feel dreadful when you do.
• If you know there's a big night out coming, use the detox supplements or advice in plans like the Pre-party Plan (see page 74) to boost your body.

The Lighten-up Plan is also good at showing you what exactly in your diet is controlling you rather than you controlling it. If you had real problems with caffeine or sugar cravings, for example, take a look at the Decaf Plan (see page 56) and the Sugar-busting Plan (see page 60) to try to tackle these specifically.

'The mistake many of us make with lunch is to pack it full of carbohydrates, like bread or jacket potatoes – too many at once can make you sleepy.'

anti-pollution plan

This plan is for anyone who lives in a big city; it's also good for anyone who truly wants to detox their body and improve their health. Pollutants are harder for the body to handle than any of the other toxins mentioned in this book, so, at some point, everyone should try this plan.

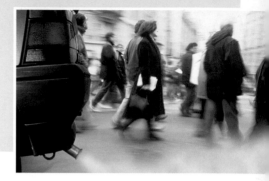

About pollutants

When you see the word 'pollution', you probably think about the brown, hazy smog that appears in the air over big cities like Los Angeles, California.

Air pollution is one of the problems that is relevant here, but it's only part of the picture. When you go on the Anti-pollution Plan, you're dealing with the effects not just of air pollution but also of the other toxins you're exposed to every day of your life. These include pesticides, additives and heavy metals in food and water; chemicals in cleaning products; gases emitted by workplace equipment like photocopiers or printers; and materials in seemingly harmless household goods like carpets, curtains and furnishings, all of which have been linked to health problems, ranging from allergies right through to cancer. It's even possible that electrical signals from your television, radio or electronic alarm clock could be polluting your body.

You may find all this hard to believe. After all, when you drink too much alcohol, eat too much sugar or mainline on caffeine for a few days, you know you're not doing

any favours to your body. The effects are obvious: you feel 'out of sorts', either sluggish or jittery, depending on your toxin of choice; your skin doesn't glow the way it should; your waistline feels puffy – sometimes you just feel poisoned. It's obvious that you need to stop taking in those things in order to feel good again, and most of us do naturally moderate our intake in such cases.

Pollutants don't work in the same way, however; most of us can't tell if we've taken in too many pesticides with our lunch, or that we've inhaled more traffic fumes than usual. But the body can tell; many pollutants create high levels of free radicals when they enter the system, and others act directly on body cells to create mutations that could become cancerous.

Strangely, when we're exposed to pollutants in the air, studies have shown that our heart rate increases, as if the body is trying to flush the toxic substance out of the system as fast as possible. Sadly, it can't actually break these chemical pollutants down. As a result, rather than keeping them in the bloodstream, the body sends toxins it can't immediately handle to be stored in the fat. In low doses, this does not cause any problems, but if high levels build up it's believed the body can become sensitive to these stored chemicals.

It is estimated, by one doctor treating this kind of illness, that at least 4 per cent of the population of the USA has some kind of chemical sensitivity, creating the common symptoms like fatigue, rashes, joint pains or headaches that most of us blame on some other element in our life.

The solution

With all this invisible pollution and chemical sensitivity in mind, you'll see that this plan is a little different from the others. While it does include a diet that will help detox your body of any pollutants in the bloodstream or liver, its main aim isn't to do this.

As stated before, the body is limited as to how it can fight toxins as potent as these. Therefore the most important part of the Anti-pollution Plan is not detoxing the pollutants but reducing your exposure to them in the first place.

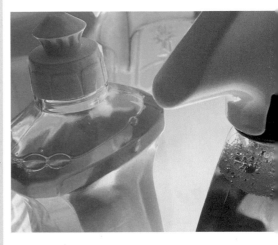

'At least 4 per cent of the US population has some kind of chemical sensitivity.'

USING GREEN CLEANERS

Many modern cleaners use large amounts of chemicals to do the job, and these can be toxic; in fact, in close proximity to each other, chlorine bleach and ammonia products can create gases that may even be fatal. Cutting down on the amount of cleaning products you use, and using them in a well-ventilated room, is vital. But it is even better to make your own green cleaners. It takes just four ingredients to clean most homes; baking soda, salt, white vinegar and lemon juice.

Air freshener. Baking soda is very good at absorbing odours. Sprinkle it onto the carpet and vacuum-clean, or just place some in pretty bowls around the house.

Furniture cleaner. One cup of lemon juice mixed with one cup of vegetable oil makes a good basic polish. Put it on the cloth rather than the furniture itself, and test on a small area first.

Window cleaner. Half-fill a spray bottle with water, then fill to the top with vinegar. Add a little washing-up liquid. Spray on the windows and wipe off.

Floor cleaner. Add half a cup of vinegar per 4.5 litres (1 gallon) of hot water, and mop as usual.

Toilet cleaner. Vinegar's dual action both kills germs and deodorizes smells. Pour one cup into your toilet bowl, leave for 10 minutes, then flush.

The three-day plan

Using the format of the normal activities of three days (a weekend and a work day), this plan points out where you are commonly exposed to toxins, and reveals how to reduce them. In some cases, it actually just takes one thing, done over this one long weekend, to make a difference to other elements of your life. This three-day plan will show you how easy it is to make changes that you can carry out from now on.

SATURDAY

7am Open your windows. The USA-based Environmental Protection Agency says that the air in the average home is two to five times more polluted than the average road. A build-up of the fumes from chemical cleaners and beauty products, like hairspray and the gas given off by mouldy walls or by synthetic material used in furniture and fabrics, is to blame, and it can cause problems like fatigue, headaches, skin rashes and allergies. Opening your windows as often as possible helps all these disperse (and is vital if you have a new carpet or furniture). It's best to do this early in the morning as pollution fumes build up outside as the day progresses.

10am Exercise safely. There's nothing better than exercising outside to boost your mood and energy – but it can also boost your exposure to airborne pollutants. After all, the average exerciser inhales ten times more air when they exercise than at rest, and breathes it into the lungs more deeply. You're also more likely to breathe through your mouth, which means air isn't passed through the tiny hairs in the nose that act as a partial filter against some pollutants.

You can help reduce risk by working out away from the rush hour (when carbon monoxide levels peak). On sunny days it may also be better to do your workout earlier in the day; sunlight increases the amount of a pollutant called ozone in the air, and this can trigger breathing problems.

11am Take your shoes off when you come back in. When researchers at the Southwest Research Institute in San Antonio in Texas, USA, analysed the carpets of homes, they found residue from pesticides sprayed up to five years earlier. These had been brought in on people's shoes and lodged within the carpet, and no amount of vacuum-cleaning could remove them. Studies have also shown that in homes where people do not routinely remove their shoes, carpets contain high levels of lead. Removing your shoes before you enter the home is normal in oriental cultures, so make it a new policy in yours.

2pm Go to the supermarket. Research carried out by the University of Ghent, Belgium, estimated that in the average daily diet a person was exposed to 54 different pesticides. You'll cut this dramatically if the weekly shop contains as much organic produce as possible. There are full details of 'going organic' on pages 15–16, but, just to remind you, the foods that will make the most difference if you swap to organic are

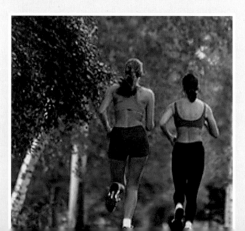

bread, milk, soft fruits, salad crops (especially lettuce), peppers, spinach, cherries, apples and peaches.

7pm When out for the evening, passive smoking is a pollutant many of us are exposed to, yet we don't realize how much it can harm us. A recent public health campaign in New Zealand estimated that one person a day died from the effects of passive smoking; their population is only 3 million people, so imagine the effects in somewhere like the UK or the USA. When you're out, try to sit in non-smoking or well-ventilated areas. Breathe through your nose, which gives some small level of filtration, rather than your mouth. If someone is blowing smoke right at you, ask them (nicely) if they can blow it the other way. If you're eating out, order something containing tomatoes: the antioxidant lycopene they contain seems to have a protective effect on the lungs, even when they are exposed to smoke.

SUNDAY
7am Get those windows open again.
10am Rearrange the furniture. Some researchers believe that the electromagnetic fields (EMFs) created by electrical appliances like televisions and radios affect the body adversely. As yet, this has not been scientifically proven, but why be sorry when being safe is so easy? EMFs don't reach more than 2–2.5m (7–8ft), so move as many electrical appliances as possible this distance away from beds, chairs or bits of the floor where you, or your children, spend plenty of time. EMF levels are highest at the rear of electrical equipment, so at the very least make sure you're not facing the back of any appliance.

2pm Green clean your home (see box on page 49).

MONDAY
7am Open the windows.
8am Simplify your beauty programme, if appropriate. It's estimated that the average woman exposes her body to 150 chemicals a day during her beauty regime, and these have been blamed for the rise in sensitive skins. Recent research has also been published that links dark hair dyes to bladder cancer. Simplify your beauty regime by using only products you really need (for example, dermatologists say that, for great skin, young women only need a cleanser, a moisturizer and sunscreen; older women can also add a vitamin C serum in the morning and a vitamin A cream in the evening). You should also try to use ranges with minimal ingredients; hypoallergenic ranges are good for this. Switch to vegetable dyes for your hair, and skip nail polishes that contain formaldehyde or toluene, both of which have been linked to serious health problems. Don't believe the hype about anti-perspirants causing breast cancer, though; it's not true.

8.30am Make your trip to work more healthy. Even though we've cleaned up our cars, traffic fumes are still our main problem when it comes to air pollution, with the rush hour offering you maximum exposure. If you drive to work, travel with your windows open and the air-conditioning off. Internal ventilation systems draw air from under the car, right by the exhaust of the car in front. It's better to drive with your windows open. This is even more important if you have a new car. Research from the Australian science researchers, CSIRO, has found toxic gases in new cars that can cause problems like headaches, skin rashes or fatigue for six months after purchase when ventilation levels in the car are low. If you walk to work, stay as far away as

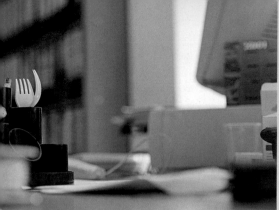

possible from the kerb, where carbon monoxide levels are at their highest, and always try to breathe through your nose not your mouth.

10am Rearrange your desk. EMFs are given off by computers and other office equipment as well as home electrical appliances, so try to avoid sitting close to anything but your computer, or next to the back of any equipment. Then add some plants to the area. Printers and photocopiers give off gases called volatile organic compounds (VOCs), which can lead to symptoms like headache, fatigue and problems with concentration. However, studies by space agency NASA have shown that spider plants, Chinese evergreens and aloe vera all filter air and can reduce the effects of VOCs. If your office has a no-plants rule, then use an air filter with a charcoal filter instead as it will help to absorb fumes.

5pm Change your clothes before you go home. This only applies if you work in an environment where toxic chemicals are used. Studies have shown that people working with toxic dusts or radioactivity can actually carry minuscule particles home on their clothes. While this doesn't cause problems to adults, it can cause a build-up in children. If you are a parent, it is best to change before you leave work.

Anti-pollution eating plan

Fighting the effects of pollutants on the body using nutrition needs a two-pronged approach. First, you can use foods called 'chelating' foods. These are foods that have the power to directly excrete toxins through the body by binding to them and carrying them out of the system (see pages 16–19). Such chelating foods include alfalfa, apples, beetroot, bananas, brussels sprouts, cabbage, carrots, cereals, garlic, onions, seaweed, tofu and watercress.

The other approach is to use antioxidant foods to fight the effects of free radicals, which are created either as the pollutants enter the body or as byproducts from those the liver does manage to break down. Antioxidant foods are those that contain the nutrients vitamin C, vitamin E, beta-carotene and selenium, plus specialist antioxidants like glutathione. Good sources include avocado, blueberries, carrots, citrus fruits, kale, kiwi fruit, prunes, pumpkin, raspberries, red grapes, red peppers, spinach, sweet potatoes, strawberries, tomatoes and watermelon.

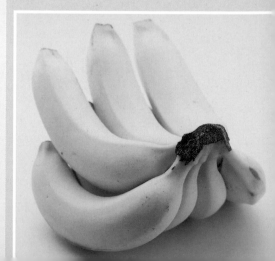

Making sure that your daily diet contains at least one chelating food and one antioxidant food in every meal will help your body to fight pollutants, but, to concentrate the effects of your programme over this long weekend, you're going to aim for considerably more than this. What follows is the three-day eating plan, including recipes.

SATURDAY

- Start the day by having an Antioxidant Smoothie for your breakfast.

Antioxidant Smoothie

2 tablespoons prepared blueberries •
2 tablespoons prepared strawberries • 250ml
(8floz) orange juice • 1 banana •
1 dessertspoonful chlorella powder
Put all the ingredients together in a blender and blend until smooth. Serve with a bowl of bran cereal topped with soya milk.

Chelating Cocktail

2–3 carrots, peeled • 1 beetroot • 1 apple
Juice all the ingredients, then serve.

Aubergine and Tofu Bake

½ aubergine, sliced • 1 teaspoon olive oil • 1 clove garlic, chopped • ½ onion, finely chopped • 1 tomato, chopped • 125g (4oz) tofu, cubed
Slice the aubergine in half lengthways. Put the pieces in a warm oven for 15 minutes, then remove and scoop out the middles, reserving the shell. Add the olive oil to a saucepan with the garlic and cook for 2–3 minutes. Mix the contents of the saucepan with the aubergine flesh. Add the tomato and tofu, and spoon it all back into the aubergine shells. Bake these in a preheated oven at 200°C (400°F) or Gas Mark 6 for about 30 minutes until they soften. Serve the stuffed aubergines shells with 2 tablespoons of cooked wholemeal pasta.

- Supplements can enhance the programme, so take these now (you should take such supplements with breakfast on the other days too). You need a multivitamin high in antioxidant nutrients and 10–12g of psyllium (take this at lunchtime too).
- Mid-morning, have a glass of Chelating Cocktail.
- For lunch, have a bowl of lentil soup, ideally a 'homemade' type of soup rather than a canned variety. Try health food stores or the chiller compartment of the supermarket for these. Serve with a salad of watercress, cherry tomatoes, red onion and avocado.
- For your evening meal, eat Aubergine and Tofu Bake.

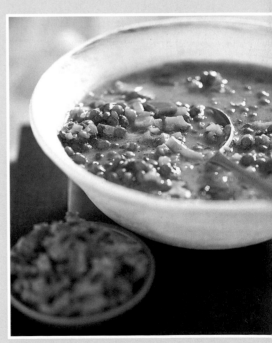

'Use antioxidant foods to fight the effects of free radicals.'

SUNDAY

- For breakfast, eat a fruit plate, made from one mango, sliced, a handful of blueberries, a banana and six prunes, served with two slices of wholemeal toast spread with honey.
- Mid-morning, have a Chelating Cocktail.
- For lunch, eat a Triple-decker Power Sandwich.
- For your evening meal, eat a grilled chicken breast served with brussels sprouts, cabbage, carrots and new potatoes, and topped with a little gravy.

MONDAY

- For breakfast, have an Antioxidant Smoothie, plus a bowl of bran cereal topped with either skimmed or soya milk.
- Mid-morning, have a Chelating Cocktail.
- For lunch, eat sushi and miso soup. Choose any selection of seaweed-covered sushi from your local supermarket or sushi bar, and serve with miso soup. You'll find this sold in health food stores or oriental supermarkets if you don't have a local sushi bar to make it for you.
- For your evening meal, eat a Mango and Avocado Salad with Smoked Chicken.

Triple-decker Power Sandwich

3 slices wholegrain bread, spread thinly with low-fat spread or low-fat mayonnaise (one piece needs covering on both sides) • handful of alfalfa sprouts • ½ avocado, sliced • 1 tomato, sliced • 1 slice of turkey • 1 slice of lean ham

Place the turkey on one slice of the wholegrain bread. Top with half the alfalfa sprouts and the avocado. Now add the slice of bread you 'buttered' on both sides. On top of this, add the lean ham, the tomato and the rest of the alfalfa. Top with the last slice of bread. Serve with a side salad of grated carrot, chopped apple and beetroot.

Mango and Avocado Salad with Smoked Chicken

handful of watercress • 25g (1oz) cooked beetroot • ½ avocado, sliced • ¼ small mango, sliced • 50g (2oz) smoked chicken, sliced • lemon juice and low-fat vinaigrette, to taste

Make up a salad of watercress and beetroot and top with the avocado and mango. Sprinkle with lemon juice and some vinaigrette dressing. Toss well, add the chicken and serve.

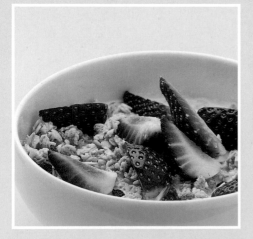

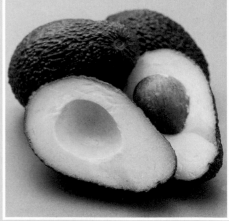

USING EXTERNAL DETOX METHODS

You can also help to detox your body from the inside by using some of the external stimulants (see pages 28–30).

Saunas – particularly those of the infrared variety – can cause the release of pollutants from fat stores. Used with the diet above, this is safe.

Another therapy commonly used by naturopaths and environmental therapists are baths of bentonite. This clay, available from health food stores, is said to draw toxins out of the body and into the water. It works because most toxins have a positive charge while clay has a negative one, so they are attracted to each other. Use one to three cups of clay in your bath.

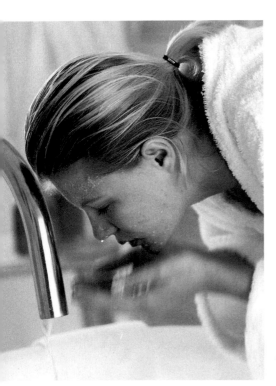

Living the detox life

In an ideal world, all the behaviours in the Anti-pollution Plan would become part of your life from now on.

Being realistic, however, if you're a busy working mum clearing up after a family every day, or a working person who can hardly face cleaning once a week, it's much easier to buy a miracle cleaner that leaves your bath sparkling in a matter of seconds than prepare your own products, no matter what the chemical cost – but not all the tips are so hard. There are 11 ways in the plan to reduce your toxic load, and some of them just mean picking up something different at the supermarket or doing something in a different way.

Even if you can keep up just half of these vital changes when the weekend is over they will start to reduce your exposure to pollutants and boost your health and wellbeing. Incorporating anti-pollutant foods or even just a glass of the Chelating Cocktail into your diet every day will help your body tackle the toxins that get thrown at it more effectively.

'Making sure that your daily diet contains at least one chelating food and one antioxidant food in every meal will help fight pollutants.'

decaf plan

If you're drinking a lot of coffee or tea, or if you're just fed up with not being able to start your day until you've had at least one cup, this is the plan for you. Caffeine is found in a lot more things than coffee and tea, however, so the Decaf Plan involves more than just cutting down on your hot beverage intake.

About caffeine

If there's one thing that keeps us working, it's caffeine. For most of us, the day doesn't begin until we've consumed at least one cup of tea or coffee, but often each cup of these we drink also comes with a big sip of guilt.

The reason is that we believe that caffeine is bad for us. We've all seen the newspaper headlines saying that it interferes with sleep, that it may decrease fertility and that it raises blood pressure – so most of us think we shouldn't drink it. But it's not strictly true. Although studies have shown the harmful effects of caffeine, they have also shown its benefits. If you drink coffee you seem to have a lower risk of gallstones, and you may have a reduced risk of developing Parkinson's disease. Caffeine can actually help the detox process, because it stimulates the bowel to move its contents along – one reason it's also been linked to a decreased risk of colon cancer.

So why is there such a contradiction? Simple. The negative studies tended to focus on intakes of over 350mg (equivalent to three to four cups of coffee) a day, while the positive results were found when people consumed less. It's clear that the idea 'all caffeine is evil' is a myth, but there is a point at which it does become toxic.

CAFFEINE TEMPTATION

This brings us to the main problem with caffeine – it's pretty easy to reach that toxic limit. Never before has caffeine been so accessible, or packaged in so many tasty treats. And coffee is only part of the picture. You can buy caffeinated yogurt, ice cream and even water. Furthermore, while five years ago no one had even heard of caffeine-rich 'energy' drinks, now the average person in Britain (where the market is largest) drinks 3.5 litres (6 pints) of these a year. The result is that 80 per cent of Britons, Americans and Australians now

Here's a guide to how much caffeine is in some common foods and drinks:

- Cup of instant coffee: 60mg
- Cup of espresso coffee: 100mg
- Cup of filter/cafetiere coffee: up to 150mg
- Cup of tea: 50mg
- Can of cola: 35–46mg, depending on brand
- Can of energy drinks: 80mg
- Small bar of milk chocolate: 15mg
- Small bar of dark chocolate: 30mg
- 250ml (8floz) chocolate milk drink: 8mg
- Painkillers: 20–100mg per pill

take in some kind of caffeine every day. What's even worse is that the more caffeine you have, the more you need.

WHY CAFFEINE IS ADDICTIVE

Caffeine's power comes from the fact that it is similar in structure to a natural substance called adenosine. This is made in the body, and is sent to the brain when the body feels that particular nerve cells are getting too active. It then binds with the cells and calms them down. However, when caffeine enters the body, it slips into the hole in the cells that adenosine would normally use. The brain cells therefore remain excited, and you stay energized. When the caffeine starts to wear off, your energy drops and, to pick yourself up again, you drink more caffeine. The more caffeine you drink the more your body gets used to it, and the more you need to get this wake-up call. What's more, if you don't take in that amount, you get withdrawal symptoms. The most common are headaches, which occur when blood vessels in the brain start to dilate (caffeine constricts them), but people can also get stomach upsets, mood swings and fatigue. After a while, the amount of caffeine you need to defend yourself against these effects gets higher, and you reach a level of caffeine where the negative effects outweigh the positive.

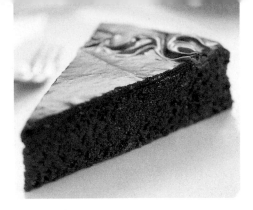

The solution

The simple way to cut down on your caffeine is to stop drinking or eating anything that contains it. That's how most detox diets work.

For some people this works perfectly; however, for at least 50 per cent of the population cutting out caffeine leads to withdrawal symptoms that can make you miserable. But giving up caffeine doesn't have to feel bad if you use this plan. The basic premise is don't come off suddenly.

Studies have shown that caffeine withdrawal doesn't occur if you cut down slowly. So, on the day you start this plan, you're going to drink whatever coffee or tea you normally do, but in every cup reduce the amount of caffeine by a quarter. So, when you pour a cup of coffee, fill a quarter of it with decaffeinated coffee. If you're drinking tea, top up with decaf; with soda, pour out a quarter of the can and refill it with a caffeine-free blend. Stick at this level for three days; if you try to cut down again before this, you could get negative symptoms. On the fourth day, cut out another quarter of a cup, and stick at this for three days. Repeat the process until you're drinking no caffeine at all per cup, which should take 12 days.

Sounds simple? Biologically it is, but there's another element of withdrawal – the mental factor. A lot of us become as dependent psychologically on caffeine as we do physically, thinking we aren't as energetic or as clear-headed without it. A sudden burst of fatigue or an urgent deadline can easily trigger a coffee craving that ruins your whole plan. Therefore, an important part of the Decaf Plan consists of preventing these triggers occurring by boosting energy levels and your brainpower.

Decaf diet

Manipulating your diet is the simplest way to avoid caffeine cravings. The most important thing you can do is eat little and often, since this keeps the blood-sugar levels constant. It also helps to cut down on sugary or refined carbohydrates (like cakes, biscuits and white bread or pasta), which send your blood-sugar levels soaring only to have them crash back down soon afterwards – a major trigger for a caffeine craving.

Instead, fill your diet with foods high in B vitamins, which your body uses to produce energy and also help you to tackle stress. Good sources of these include wholegrain foods like brown rice or bread, breakfast cereals and some fruits and vegetables, including asparagus and bananas. These are also good because they boost fibre levels in your body: the fibre takes over from the caffeine as a bowel stimulator.

However, don't eat just carbohydrates and vegetables. B vitamins are also found in dairy products, meat and poultry, which provide the body with protein. Protein takes longer than carbohydrates to break down, which helps normalize blood-sugar levels.

Finally, drink plenty of water. If the ideal amount of water in your body falls by 3 per cent you'll start feeling fatigued and your brain will function up to 10 per cent more slowly; so drink at least one glass of water an hour. Here's a suggested eating plan, with recipes.

Breakfast
- Glass of Energy Juice.
- Bowl of a bran or wheat cereal with skimmed milk, topped with a chopped banana.

Energy Juice
2 apples • 1 peach • 1 orange • 2.5cm (1in) cube of ginger root
Juice all the ingredients, and then serve.

- Cup of coffee, one-quarter filled with a decaffeinated brand (always drink this instead of normal coffee).

Mid-morning snack
- A handful of dried apricots chopped and mixed into some low-fat cottage cheese.
- Cup of ginger tea, or another glass of Energy Juice.

Lunch
- 75g (3oz) of sliced chicken on top of an energizing salad of baby spinach, red pepper, broccoli florets, cherry tomatoes and grated carrot. Serve with a bowl of vegetable or lentil soup.
- Take a ginkgo supplement to deflect the natural dip in energy and mental clarity that occurs after lunch.

Mid-afternoon snack
- Mix proteins and carbohydrates quickly and easily with a little grated low-fat cheese on rye crispbread, and throw in some energizing vitamins by topping it with slices of beetroot and tomato.

Evening meal
- Keep things simple with a 75g (3oz) grilled salmon steak served with a brown rice, red onion and asparagus salad and a side serving of green beans.

Before bed
- Have a glass of warm milk to keep your energy stable overnight and to aid sleep.

ENERGIZING BODY AND MIND

You can also use alternative therapies, supplements and homeopathic remedies to energize your body and your mind.

- Use the power of aromatherapy; sprinkle three to four drops of an energizing oil like lime, lemon or grapefruit onto a tissue and then inhale.
- Equally easy is stimulating one of the acupressure points on the wrist. Look for the crease closest to your palm and press the area of this directly under your thumb 5–10 times.
- If you need a kick from a cup, try coffee substitutes like chicory and barley, or ginger tea. Alternatively, try drinking some Energy Juice (see opposite).
- Breathing exercises will also help. According to experts, the best way to energize the body is with explosions of breath, to cleanse the lungs of old air. Open your mouth wide, inhale deeply, then let the breath out with a big 'Hah'. Repeat this process for 30 seconds.
- It may help to take ginkgo biloba. In research carried out by the University of Northumberland in the UK, this helped boost people's mental energy and concentration after just one dose. The best time to take it is probably just after lunch; we have a natural energy dip mid-afternoon, which your lunchtime supplement will counteract.
- The advice in this plan should make giving up caffeine symptom-free. However, if you have been drinking very high doses or use coffee as a crutch, you might suffer withdrawal headaches. If this happens, try the homeopathic remedy coffea crudea.

Living the detox life

After the 12 days you've been on the plan, you should be completely caffeine-free. At this point, don't jump straight back into a cup or two a day. Instead, try to manage for at least two weeks without caffeine so you can retrain the way you think about it and the role it plays in your life.

Once you've done that, if you want to start drinking caffeine again, go ahead; after all, it could actually help your health. But, to live the decaf life to the full, stick to the following rules:

- Keep your caffeine intake under 300mg a day (roughly three 180ml (6floz) cups of coffee), or if you do drink more, don't do it for more than two days.
- You'll take less caffeine in with your coffee if you drink instant (it contains 60mg per 180ml (6floz) cup, compared to a small espresso, containing 100mg in a 60ml (2floz) cup). Drip-brewed or filter coffee is the most potent – 150mg per 180ml (6floz).
- Don't forget that coffee isn't the only caffeine-containing food. Don't add to your intake with tea, chocolate, soft drinks or even headache pills.
- Don't rely on caffeine-containing drinks and foods to perk you up. Use the energizing suggestions in the box, or just go outside and get some fresh air. The less you feel you 'need' coffee, the less you'll actually drink.

sugar-busting plan

This is the plan to use if you like sugar a lot, if your day simply isn't complete without a couple of chocolate bars, if you regularly crave sugary foods or drinks or if you just use sugary foods to fuel your day's energy dips and would like to stop.

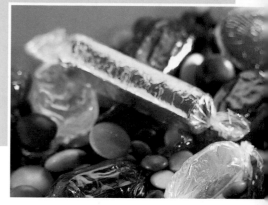

About sugar

If you're a sugar addict, you're not alone. House-hold surveys in the US and Britain have found that the average American citizen eats 30kg (64lb) of sugar a year, while Britons each eat 9kg (20lb).

In France, eating cakes is seen as one of the best ways to make yourself happy (53 per cent of the population say they do it), and 36 per cent of Europeans eat chocolate to deal with stress. It may even be programmed into us to like sugar; it's well known that babies actually taste amniotic fluid in the womb, and when scientists put sugary substances into that fluid they taste it a lot more often.

There's a lot about sugar to like. It boosts your mood by producing the happy hormone serotonin in the brain, it can provide a temporary energy boost and it tends to come wrapped up in tasty treats like chocolate, cakes or ice cream. When you're feeling down or fatigued, or even feeling like you did a great thing today and you need a treat, reaching for something sugary is a natural and happy reaction, and a lot cheaper than retail therapy.

Therefore, bearing all this in mind, the following is not going to be good news: most of us do need to cut down our intake. The truth is that sugar is rapidly shaping up to be one of the major food toxins, with researchers at the New York State University in Buffalo, USA, recently naming it the number one ageing food. Other health experts claim it's one of the major promoters of poor health in the 21st century. There are a few reasons for this:

1 Sugar increases the levels of toxic free radicals. In fact, eating 300g (10½oz) of sugar boosts free radical numbers by 140 per cent.

2 Sugar affects immunity. When it needs to, the average white blood cell can gobble up about 14 germs in an hour (someone really has measured this), but when exposed to 100g (3½oz) of sugar this number falls to only 1.4 germs, and, furthermore, stays that way for two hours.

Tackling sugar overload is therefore something that should be part of any good detox plan. But this doesn't mean living a life without any of the sweet stuff.

According to the US Department of Agriculture, a safe level of sugar is about 40g (1½oz) a day. If you can reduce your intake to this, or below, you'll dramatically improve your health. In fact, you'll have more energy than ever before, you'll be ill less often, you'll find it easier to control your weight and your skin will be less likely to get wrinkles. Convinced? Here's how to get started.

The solution

The first step in cutting sugar out of your diet is identifying exactly where it appears in your diet.

Only 30 per cent of the sugar we eat is actually in the form of obviously sugary foods such as chocolate, sweets or sugary drinks. The rest comes from hidden sugars in other foods like low-fat yogurt (a normal serving contains around 8g or ¼oz), baked beans (an average can contains around 30g or 1oz) or a glass of orange juice (around 20g or ¾oz).

Your first step in the Sugar-busting Plan is to identify the high-sugar foods in your diet by checking the labels for a figure for added sugars. Anything over about 20g a serving is a high-sugar food. If sugar isn't indicated, check the ingredient list; sugar hides under many names, including sucrose, dextrose, maltose, glucose (in fact anything ending in 'ose'), inverted syrup, corn syrup and malt extract. If any of these appear in the first three ingredients, or if more than two appear in any one food, it probably contains too much sugar. For the next two weeks, all of these foods will go from your diet (while you're trying to break the sugar cycle you need to abstain from them). The reason for this is that our

SUGAR AND ENERGY
The most immediate problem with sugar is the effect it has on our energy:

• Sugar is absorbed rapidly into the bloodstream.
• This sudden rush panics the body and a higher than normal amount of insulin (the hormone that creates energy from food) is released.
• The insulin quickly moves the sugar out of the bloodstream, leaving the body without any accessible fuel.
• You feel tired, which sends the body into panic again as it needs fuel fast. It knows that last time it ate sugar it got a surge of energy, so it stimulates the brain to start craving sugar.

This becomes a vicious circle, and one that gradually ends up with us taking in much more sugar than is good for us.

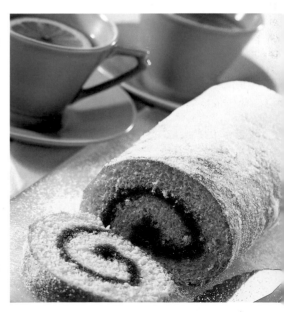

tastebuds are very attuned to sugar; the more of it they taste the more they like it. But if you can abstain from sugar for ten days (the time it takes to adjust your tastebuds to any new taste), they will be less dependent. When you do eat sugar again, you'll need much less of it to get those pleasurable sensations, which will help keep your levels down.

WHAT TO EAT

When you've removed all those sugar-filled foods from your diet, what are you going to eat? If you have read the Decaf Plan (see page 56), you'll know that diet is the key. If you've been sucked into the sugar spiral, reducing levels will lead to drops in energy while you rebalance things. You may also find your mood drops as you're no longer receiving those extra bursts of serotonin. However, by eating correctly you can counteract these things, and make the whole process so much easier on your body and mind. Here is what to eat instead:

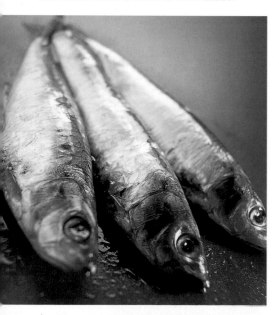

Unrefined carbohydrates. It's not just sugar that boosts serotonin in the brain – all carbohydrates do. Therefore, eating plenty of starchy foods will boost your mood and decrease stress, but it's important to eat the right type. Refined carbohydrates like white bread, white pasta and white rice cause almost as high a surge in blood sugar as sugary foods do, so basing your new eating plan around these will actually stimulate sugar cravings. Instead, you should be aiming to eat starchy foods that cause a slow increase in blood sugar (also known as foods with a low glycaemic index, or GI). The best of these include lentils, kidney beans, wholemeal pasta, plain bran cereals, sweet potatoes, brown rice, new potatoes, rye bread, pumpernickel bread, oatmeal and chickpeas.

Chicken and dairy products. These are protein foods; not only does protein keep blood-sugar levels stable but it also boosts levels of other chemicals in the brain that help reinforce mood and energy. In fact, it's been shown that within just 30 minutes of eating 75–125g (3–4oz) of a protein food such as fish, chicken, dairy products and beans people feel more energized, alert and assertive.

Fish. As well as being a protein food and therefore offering all the benefits described above, fish has a special role to play. The job of keeping brain cells receptive to the positive benefits of mood-enhancers like serotonin falls to substances called omega-3 fatty acids, which are primarily found in fish and shellfish. No wonder Finnish researchers found once-a-week fish-eaters were 31 per cent less likely to feel depressed than those who skipped fish totally.

Snacks. Eating little and often is vital to the success of the Sugar-busting Plan, because it keeps the blood-sugar levels more stable than eating three big meals a day does.

For best results, snacks should also be low-GI foods. Some of the best are cherries, grapefruit, nuts, dried apricots, low-fat yogurt, pears, apples, plums and popcorn. Proteins such as cottage cheese, tuna, nuts and seeds are also good.

WHAT NOT TO EAT OR DRINK

Refined carbohydrates. As stated above, these can cause sudden rushes in the blood-sugar levels that can trigger a sugar craving.
Caffeine. For exactly the same reason, if giving up coffee and sugar at the same time is too tough, at least eat a protein snack with your coffee to try to reduce the likelihood of a sudden sugar surge.
Alcohol. This is a sugar, and so it can trigger sugar cravings.
Artificial sweeteners. These don't raise insulin levels, but studies have shown that they may make you want to eat more. If you're feeling unsatisfied, you'll be more likely to grab a sugar-filled snack.

'When you've removed all those sugar-filled foods from your diet, what are you going to eat?'

Suggested eating plan

So what does this look like on the plate? Here are enough breakfasts, lunches and dinners to keep you going for a week. Mix and match them over two weeks, and by the end of it you'll find you are sugar-free.

Breakfasts

- A bowl of bran flakes with skimmed or soya milk accompanied by a handful of cherries.
- Two slices of rye bread topped with peanut butter followed by half a grapefruit.
- Fruit yogurt topped with dried apricots.
- Baked apple topped with a carton of natural yogurt.
- Boiled egg served with two slices of pumpernickel toast.
- A bowl of porridge topped with a small amount of chopped apple.
- Smoked kipper with some grilled tomatoes.

Lunches

- An open sandwich of tuna on rye, pumpernickel or wholegrain bread topped with alfalfa sprouts, sliced tomatoes and cucumber. Serve this with a cup of lentil soup.
- Chicken salad (grilled chicken with rocket, red peppers, red onions and celery).
- Vegetable chilli, heavy on the kidney beans and served with or without brown rice.
- Hummus served with crudités as well as a cup of tomato soup.
- Poached eggs on toast, with two slices of lean ham and a dash of hollandaise sauce.
- Slices of turkey, served with new potato salad, beetroot, grated carrot and lettuce.
- Baked beans on rye toast, topped with a generous serving of grated cheese.

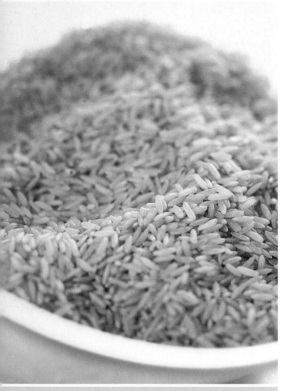

WHAT TO DO IF CRAVINGS STRIKE

While this suggested eating plan should kill off all your sugar cravings, some people will still develop the odd urge for something sweet. Here's what to do if, one day, that happens to you.

Take some rhodiola. This is available from health food stores. Used extensively in Russia, this herb is from a family called the adaptogens, which help balance your body against stress fatigue. In trials, it has been shown to increase levels of serotonin in the brain by 30 per cent and to balance blood-sugar levels.

Do some exercise. Ten minutes of exercise at a moderate rate (until you are slightly out of breath) are enough to improve both your mood and your energy levels. If a sugar craving strikes, go out for a walk.

Sniff some vanilla. Studies at St George's Hospital in London have shown that the scent of vanilla reduces sugar cravings.

Eat something. If you really are desperate to have a sweet snack, then eat something. One piece of chocolate does not break a diet – only the second one does that!

Try taking gymnema sylvestre. This is available from health food stores. It is the right supplement for you if you're actually giving in to sugar cravings. Known as the 'sugar destroyer' in Indian medicine, it acts on the tastebuds that normally detect sugar and make it tasteless. The effects last about two hours, so it's best used if you know that cravings usually come at a certain point in the day. Try drinking one cup of the tea or take one 100mg supplement.

Evening meals

- Grilled salmon steak, served with a selection of vegetables and new potatoes.
- Tomato and seafood sauce, served with a portion of wholemeal spaghetti.
- Tofu, vegetable and cashew nut stir-fry accompanied by brown rice.
- Tandoori chicken with dhal.
- Lean roast beef, a selection of vegetables and roast sweet potatoes.
- Vegetable and prawn kebabs accompanied by brown rice.
- Wholemeal spaghetti topped with some carbonara sauce.

Living the detox life

So you've finished the plan and you're sugar-free – now what? How do you live a low-sugar life? Here are some easy-to-follow guidelines.

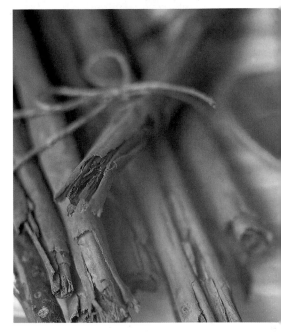

- Stick to the 40g (1½oz) rule. Once you come off the Sugar-busting Plan, it's all right to introduce sugar again, but try not to go over this amount per day. Eat non-processed foods where possible and, if you do eat canned or ready prepared foods choose no-added-sugar brands. After all, what would you rather spend your reduced sugar allowance on – a crème brûlée, or a can of baked beans and some ketchup?
- Keep refined carbohydrate levels as low as possible. This can help stop the blood-sugar swings that can trigger cravings for fast-fix sugars.
- Know your sugar substitutes. The flavours of some herbs and spices can reduce the need for sugar. In recipes, reduce the amount of sugar used by half by adding a little nutmeg, vanilla or cinnamon to take its place. Cinnamon can reduce tartness in an apple pie, for example.
- Don't eat sugar on an empty stomach. Grabbing a chocolate bar at 3pm or knocking back a doughnut for breakfast is going to cause a bigger sugar rush (and fall) than eating sugar with other foods, as in the latter case insulin will have other foods to tackle as well. If you really want something sweet, make sure you eat sugar as part of a meal or as a dessert.
- If you do have a major sugar binge, you can reduce the damage caused. The antioxidant alpha lipoic acid is known as being 'anti-sugar', because it actually stops sugar attaching to proteins in the body. It is found within foods such as broccoli, spinach, red meat and liver so make sure you eat these regularly.

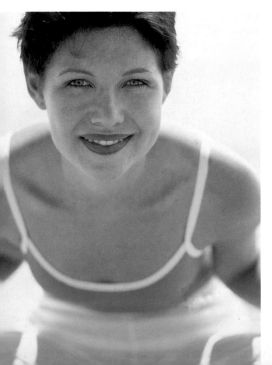

stress-busting plan

Although some degree of stress is good for us, we've all had points in our life when stress has overwhelmed us and become a toxin. Sometimes it's for a couple of days; other times it's over weeks or even months. The next time this happens to you, use this plan to help detox the damage.

About stress

Most of us think that stress is a modern-day phenomenon, caused by our longer working weeks or our need to juggle home and career. But that's not strictly true.

While the type of stress we are tackling now may be uniquely of the 21st century, stress has been felt by our ancestors since early times, and it's always been dealt with in the same way. When you start to feel that buzzing sensation that tells you something is starting to stress you, you're drawing on techniques developed by your species centuries ago to handle it.

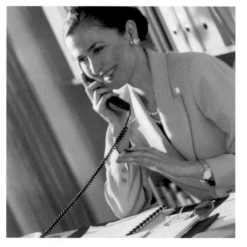

When something stresses us, the hypothalamus in the brain tells glands called the adrenals to start producing stress hormones. There are many of these hormones (adrenaline and cortisol being two of the best known) and they lead to a cascade of reactions in the body. For example, the pupils dilate, the immune system starts to release white blood cells and the heart begins to pump more rapidly, sending blood surging to the arms and legs. You breathe faster in order to flood this blood with oxygen, and your muscles tense.

WHY WE GET STRESSED

The reason all this happens is that back in our primitive days when we encountered stress it tended to be something dangerous. We had two ways to handle it: stay and fight, or run away. The physical activity involved burned up all the chemicals the stress reaction released so when the fight or the running was over, the stress was gone and there were no after-effects.

This can also happen in modern life. We may not run away from the deadline that's stressing us, or fight the boss but if something stresses us we handle it, making all those reactions calm down and go, leaving us unscathed (and probably feeling pretty good). Often what happens, however, is that as soon as we tackle one stressful thing another one hits us. Sometimes we don't even have the time to tackle the original stressor, and others build up on top of it. Over and over again, we trigger the stress reaction without letting it settle down. When this happens, stress becomes a toxin.

WHY STRESS IS TOXIC

Too much stress means that all those positive actions that fire us up to deal with our stressors start to turn on our body. Our increased heart rate begins to put pressure on the heart, fatiguing it and potentially increasing the risk of heart attack. The muscles that have tensed begin to spasm, which leads to problems like backache and headache. Those white blood cells that were released in case we got wounded have nowhere to go, and these can trigger allergies and aggravate auto-immune diseases like arthritis. Finally, after a stretch of pumping out all these chemicals, the adrenal glands start to fatigue, and so do we. Beating stress is therefore a vital way to help our health.

The solution

This plan is probably the simplest to follow in the book. There are ten simple techniques that will help you reduce stress physically and mentally, or that will help strengthen your body against it.

When you're stressed, the last thing you need to be doing is feeling you have to follow a strict and regimented plan; trying to follow such a regime could even add to your tension load. Instead, next time you're stressed, or if you know stress is coming and want to strengthen your body against it, just turn to this plan and use two or three of the following techniques each day.

Top 10 stress fighters

1 **PLANNING YOUR LIFE**
The most important way to detox stress at work is to manage your time and your duties. When you get to your desk, spend 10 minutes deciding what needs doing, and in what order. It's believed that you get a fifth more work done each day if you do this, and you do the work better. When researchers looked at students in Seneca College in Toronto, Canada, they found that students who planned their work were much more likely to have A and B grades than those who didn't plan things. It's also vital to say no to things you don't have time to do: nothing creates stress more than overloading yourself, and learning to say no is a vital aid to beating its effects. This may sound simple, but if you just do these two things you'll dramatically lower your stress load.

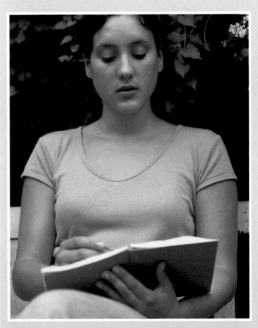

2 CUTTING DOWN ON CAFFEINE

Caffeine stimulates the adrenal glands to produce stress hormones, and research at

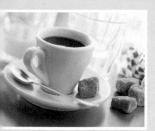

the USA's Duke University showed that four to five cups of coffee a day boosted levels of stress hormones by up to a third. Stick to one to two cups a day, or get your lift from ginger or peppermint teas, which boost energy and mental clarity without creating stress reactions. (See also the Decaf Plan on page 56.)

3 PRACTISING YOGA

When doctors at the USA's Roosevelt Hospital measured people's stress scores after 25 minutes of yoga, they found that tension levels had dramatically decreased. Other studies have shown that yoga can decrease blood pressure in a matter of minutes. This all combines to make yoga an important part of stress management. There are many yoga postures that help to relieve stress, but, when it comes to an all-round stress-busting package, the 'Salute to the Sun' (see opposite) can't be beaten. It's an instant energizer – so much so that it should only be done in the morning. It releases tensions in the muscles, stimulates the circulation and lymphatic system and, by allowing you to focus on your body and take time out, it helps reduce the mental toll of stress. Finally, through using upward and downward movements, it aims to strengthen and balance the adrenal glands. The postures are described step by step, but you should aim to perform them as one long fluid series of moves.

4 B VITAMINS

As is the case with all the detox plans in this book, what you eat is vitally important to the success of the programme. When it comes to fighting stress, you want to focus on the B vitamins that help support the adrenal glands and give you energy. Good sources of B vitamins include breakfast cereals, wholegrain bread, milk, meat, yogurt, eggs, bananas and dried fruits. You should therefore try to include some of these in every meal.

5 RELEASING TENSION THROUGHOUT THE DAY

When we're under stress, many of us hold our body in unusual or uncomfortable positions without realizing that we are doing so. This can cause a lot of muscular tension, and result in aches in the head or back. Doing some simple stretching exercises at your desk can therefore help (see below).

Stretching exercises

- Sitting straight, shrug your shoulders up towards your ears. As you go up, tense all the muscles then release them on the way down. Repeat 4–5 times.
- Interlock your fingers and, turning your palms to face outwards, straighten your arms out in front of you. Push gently forward so you feel the stretch along your shoulder blades. Hold for 10 seconds.
- Keeping your fingers interlocked, push your arms up above your head and stretch your torso upwards. Hold for 10 seconds.
- Finally, tip your head gently to one side so you feel a stretch on the side of your neck. Hold for 10 seconds. Bring your head back to the centre, then tip it to the other side and hold for 10 seconds again.

'SALUTE TO THE SUN' EXERCISE

- **1** Stand up straight with the palms of your hands together in front of your chest (as if praying). Breathe regularly. Inhale, then raise your arms straight up above your head and carefully bend backwards from the waist a few centimetres until you feel a stretch across the whole of your front.

- **2** Exhale, then bend forwards from your hip joints. Place your hands on the floor on either side of your feet (at first you will need to bend your knees to do this, but gradually you will become more flexible). Inhale and look up. As you do this, place your left foot behind you as far as you can. Step back with your right foot so the weight of your body is carried by your hands and feet. Your body should make a straight line from your hands to your feet.

- **3** Exhale and lower your knees to the floor. Then lower your chest and chin.

- **4** Inhaling, lower your body so you are lying flat. Now slowly arch your back from the waist so your chest comes off the floor. Your hands should stay on the floor but your arms will straighten.

- **5** Exhale, bend your knees, then straighten your arms and legs and push your hips up to make an inverted V. Inhale and step between your hands with your left foot. Exhale, then step up with your right foot. Now, slowly and while inhaling, bring yourself up to the standing position.

Repeat the sequence from step 2 onwards as many times as you like (it takes about 5 minutes to do 20 sequences). Remember to alternate the leading foot in the step 2. The faster you carry out 'Salute to the Sun' the more energizing it is, but get to know the moves before speeding up.

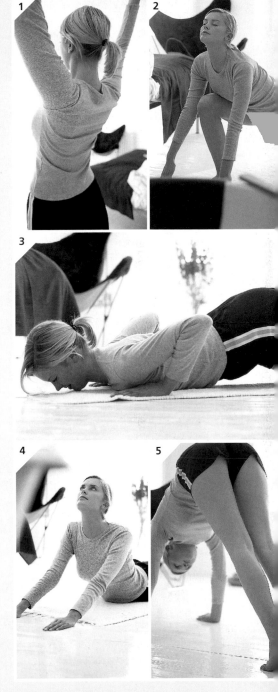

6 EATING CARBOHYDRATES FOR LUNCH

According to Dr Judith Wurtman, one of the world's leading authorities on food and mood, and her team at the Massachusetts Institute of Technology, USA, the ultimate calming lunch is one based on carbohydrate foods, which boost levels of the hormone serotonin in the brain. However, it doesn't take a whole plate of pasta for this to happen; eating too many carbohydrates in one go can actually make you sleepy and lethargic. Instead, the best carbohydrate dose is 40–50g (1½–2oz) of a starchy carbohydrate like bread, pasta, rice or potato. Serve this with a big side salad or some steamed vegetables to fill you up. Sadly, you can't add protein, since this dulls the calming effect. If you get hungry later in the afternoon, you can snack on a few handfuls of low-fat popcorn or some rice cakes with some fruit – these will take the edge off your hunger but will also refuel your bank of calming chemicals.

7 EXERCISE

If you want to reduce your stress symptoms by a third, work out when you're under pressure. Clinical trials have found that exercise reduces stress by burning off the excess adrenaline produced by the adrenal glands. It takes just 10 minutes of activity to start this process and boost mood – even walking can have the desired effect.

8 USING A SCENTED STRESS DETOXER

Beating stress is one of the major uses for aromatherapy and it works in a number of different ways. The oils calm us psychologically, reduce tension in the muscles and can strengthen the adrenal glands. A great stress-beating blend is two drops of lavender, two drops of mandarin and one drop of jasmine oil. Either add these to 10ml (⅓floz) of carrier oil and ask someone to apply them via the back massage given on pages 32–33, or use it yourself as part of the neck and shoulder massage described on page 31. Alternatively, put the blend in the bath, sit back and relax for 15 minutes. Don't, however, use the blend if you are pregnant – instead you should use mandarin oil, which is safe for pregnant women.

9 SUPPLEMENTING YOUR ADRENAL GLANDS

There are many herbs that can help do this, but one of the most commonly used by herbalists is ginseng. Ginseng is an adaptogenic herb: this means it helps the body balance itself in times of physical and mental stress. As yet, no one knows exactly why, but research seems to indicate that it acts on the hypothalamus, controlling its messages to the adrenal glands and reducing the amount of stress hormones produced. The recommended dose of ginseng is 500–1000mg a day, and it's best taken before food. Also, don't take ginseng

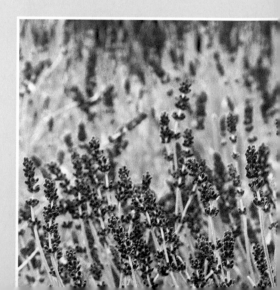

for more than three weeks without a break as it loses its effectiveness if taken for extended periods of time.

10 PLANNING FOR A GOOD NIGHT'S SLEEP

If you are tired, your ability to handle stress is compromised. When you're stressed, however, it can be hard to switch off to sleep, which is why you should start preparing for sleep about two hours before you go to bed, with your evening meal. A number of foods have calming and sedating properties, and so by including these in your evening meal you can wind your body down from the day. The best foods to choose include:

Lettuce. This contains lactucarium, which is a natural sedative.

Red onions. The antioxidant quercetin they contain is calming.

Milk or dairy products. They contain natural opiates called casomorphins.

Starchy carbohydrates. Brown rice, pasta or potatoes, which create serotonin.

A little protein. This contains an ingredient called tryptophan, which is also used to create serotonin.

5-minute fixes

By using all the techniques in the plan, your stress load should dramatically reduce. However, if you do feel yourself starting to tense, it's good to try to get things under control as quickly as possible. Here are some 5-minute fixes that will lower your arousal level.

- Calm your breath. Inhaling through your nose to a count of 5 and exhaling through your mouth to a count of 10 instantly calms the body.
- Suck half a teaspoon of honey. This takes just 5 minutes to stimulate serotonin in the brain.
- Warm your hands. When we are stressed, our hands cool, but warming them (simply try sitting on them) lowers stress.
- The Bach flower remedy 'Rescue Remedy' (available from health food stores) fortifies the body quickly, and is particularly good for shock.
- Stimulate the de-stressing acupressure point in your feet. Find the furrow on the top of your foot where the bones of your first and second toes meet. Then gently press this 10 times.

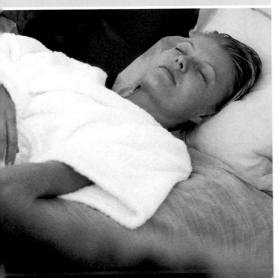

'When you're stressed it can be hard to switch off to sleep, which is why you should start preparing for sleep about two hours before you go to bed.'

One day to de-stress

Looking at all the above, you may find it hard to pick two or three things that will do you the most good. That's not a problem, since you can actually fit them all into one working day – even a really busy one, if you focus. Here's what you should do.

7am Take 5 minutes for the 'Salute to the Sun' yoga exercise (see page 69).

7.15am Take your ginseng supplement.

7.30am Have breakfast. Use this as a time to boost your B vitamins. A bowl of breakfast cereal topped with skimmed milk, a chopped banana and a handful of raisins is a good choice. Alternatively try poached eggs on toast with a glass of milk and a handful of dried apricots.

9am Get to work and spend ten minutes planning your day and clearing your desk.

11am Have a calming carbohydrate snack (like rice cakes and fruit).

1pm Have lunch. Remember to focus on carbohydrates at this point in the day: jacket potato and salad is a good choice.

1.30pm Go for a half-hour walk outside. The activity and the fresh air will help reduce tension and energize you.

3pm Take a 5-minute stretch break at your desk to wipe out tension.

7pm Back at home, conjure up a calming evening meal, such as Calming Chicken Fajitas.

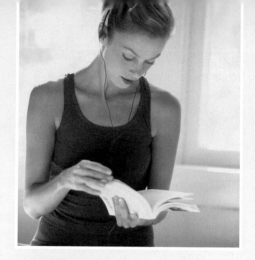

9pm Have a calming detox bath or massage.

10pm Go to bed for a great night's sleep.

Calming Chicken Fajitas (serves two)

2 teaspoons olive oil • 175g (6oz) chicken, cut into strips • ½ red onion, sliced • ½ red pepper, sliced • ½ yellow pepper, sliced • 2 tablespoons salsa • 50g (2oz) lettuce, chopped finely • 50g (2oz) grated cheese • 4 wholewheat tortilla sheets • 50g (2oz) (dry weight) brown rice, cooked

Heat the oil in a frying pan and then add the chicken. Stir-fry for 2 minutes, then add the onion and peppers. Keep frying until the chicken is cooked through and the onion and peppers have softened. In the meantime, take the tortilla sheets and spread these with the salsa (divided equally between them). Leaving 2.5cm (1in) at the bottom of each sheet and 2.5cm (1in) to the right, fill them with a quarter of the lettuce and grated cheese. Now top each with the chicken, onion and peppers. Fold the unfilled 2.5cm (1in) of each tortilla over the filling, then roll over to the right until 'sealed'. Serve with the rice.

Living the detox life

While this programme will help you beat stress when it happens, it's actually better for your health if you can try to reduce stress at the source – before it happens. The following methods will help you to tackle the first signs:

- Do a stress audit. For one month, look at the most common things in your life that stress you, and find ways to tackle them. This could be as simple as fixing a hook by the front door so you don't spend 10 minutes each morning trying to find your keys; or something 'serious' like telling your boss you can't handle that extra project this month after all.
- Keep your arousal level low. If you start feeling stressed, don't panic. Stress is like a tower of cards; you're fine until you put the one thing on top that sends it toppling. If you begin to feel stressed, tackle some of the simple things that are adding to the problem, such as a phone call you need to make, or ask the kids to play outside for 10 minutes to give you some space. If you remove the little stressors, the big one won't feel as bad.
- Write down your worries. This works in two ways. Writing down what you're worried about can help you prioritize what you can deal with so that you can get it out of your head. What's left should be subjected to a perception audit. Write down everything that's stressing you. Now think what the worst thing that could happen with the problem is. Out of ten, how likely is it that the worst will happen? If it's less than six, forget it. If it's more, stop worrying about it and start thinking of ways to solve the problem: positive planning is a great way to reduce stress.

'Look at the most common things in your life that stress you, and find ways to tackle them.'

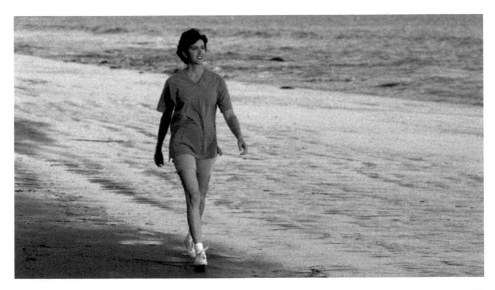

pre-party plan

Over-indulgence in alcohol can cause serious damage to the body, but in the real world most people enjoy a drink. This plan is therefore not going to tell you how to give up alcohol completely; instead it's going to show you how to protect your body against the damage that alcohol can cause.

About alcohol

Traditional detox books would probably say that all alcohol is evil and that it must never pass your lips again.

But that's simply not true. A small amount of alcohol is positively good for you. Studies of 19,500 Spanish adults found that people who drank moderate amounts of alcohol had less incidence of sickness than teetotallers, and felt healthier and happier about their bodies. Wine has been shown to help reduce arthritis symptoms, and may also help ward off cancer because of antioxidants found in the grapes.

The highest protective effect, however, is in the cardiovascular system, because alcohol helps thin the blood, reducing the risk of clotting and arterial furring; it also increases levels of a protective form of cholesterol called high-density lipoproteins (HDLs). So people who have one or two drinks a day live longer than those who don't.

ALCOHOL BACKLOG

However, if those one or two drinks turn into three or more, the protective effects stop and alcohol starts to attack. It triggers a rise in levels of fats called triglycerides (which promote arterial furring) in the blood. On top of this, the body's blood vessels dilate, so the heart has to pump faster to circulate blood around the body, putting pressure on it. Instead of the antioxidants in alcohol fighting cancer, high levels can actually cause mutations in cells that may trigger disease (see the box opposite). In fact, excess alcohol has a detrimental effect on just about all the body's systems. When alcohol enters, the body turns all its resources into getting rid of it. Unfortunately, it can only handle one drink an hour. More than this and a backlog builds up, stressing and damaging the liver and resulting in a hangover. The Pre-party Plan works by strengthening your body against the effects alcohol has, reducing those unpleasant feelings the next day.

TOO MUCH OF A GOOD THING

Occasionally indulging in a couple of drinks poses no problem to your body. The alcohol will pass through your system leaving it unscathed. If you imbibe more than three drinks in a night, however, the body goes into minor panic.

- This starts in the stomach, where it triggers an immune response designed to attack the 'poison'. Part of this is the release of histamine, which can actually irritate the stomach lining – leading to pain and nausea.
- The stomach stops absorbing substances from food (probably to try to slow alcohol absorption). This prevents the absorption of vital vitamins and nutrients needed to fight the alcohol and keep you well. In fact, one US study showed that heavy drinkers needed to take six times more vitamin C than non-drinkers to end up with the same amounts in their body.
- In the liver, alcohol is broken down into a substance called acetaldehyde. This attacks the fibres that hold your skin together and leads to wrinkles. It also alters the shape of red blood cells, causing lower blood oxygen levels, and attacks normal cells, creating mutations that may become cancerous.
- Alcohol switches off the hormone that helps the body retain water, leading to dehydration and headaches.

The solution

The most important thing you can do to prepare your body for alcohol is to ensure your liver is in fine fighting form – after all, you're relying on its strength to process alcohol out of your system quickly and cleanly.

Top of your list of weapons here should be milk thistle (see page 39), which strengthens the outer membranes of liver cells, protecting them from damage caused by alcohol and prolonging the time at which they work at full power. In informal studies at the Integrative Medicine Medicinal Group at Cedars-Sinai Medical Centre in Los Angeles, USA, hangover symptoms were reduced in student volunteers taking milk thistle in the days before a big end-of-term party. However, you should also take a supplement called N-Acetyl-Cysteine. This contains a mix of amino acids including one called cysteine, which in the body converts into the vital detox enzyme glutathione – this acts directly on the metabolism of alcohol. A study published in New Scientist magazine found that it prevented hangover symptoms completely.

You also need to get your nutrient stores in shape. The body uses masses of nutrients when it is processing alcohol: one nutrient niacin (or vitamin B3), for example, binds to the acetaldehyde molecule, transporting it out of the system. If your levels of B3 are low, this process will be

'The plan works by strengthening your body against the effects alcohol has upon it, and therefore reducing those unpleasant hangover feelings the next day.'

impaired and alcohol can stay in the system for longer. Loading up on foods containing high levels of the B vitamins (as all of this essential group help metabolize alcohol), such as wholegrain bread, breakfast cereal, meat and leafy green vegetables, is therefore a vital part of the Pre-party Plan. You should also aim to maximize your intake of vitamin C, which is destroyed by alcohol but which helps fight the cellular damage it causes. Aim for around 500mg during the day; to get this high amount, the best sources are kiwi fruit, blueberries and red peppers. You also need adequate supplies of zinc, which helps the B vitamins do their job, and is contained in red meat, poultry and wholegrains.

Lastly, you need to prepare your body to take in alcohol. If you are going on a binge, line your stomach. It's not a myth: if you eat before you leave home, you will be able to handle your alcohol more effectively than if you drink on an empty stomach. In fact, a study in the *Journal of Forensic Science* showed that, if you eat a meal with fat, protein and carbohydrates in it, you absorb alcohol three times more slowly than on an empty stomach.

Putting the plan into practice

So that's what to do, and now here's how to do it. This plan can be used during the day before any evening party, but it will bring much better results if you stick to it for two or three days before you plan to drink.

Morning

- Take 200mg of milk thistle.
- Breakfast on a bran cereal topped with skimmed milk and two tablespoons of blueberries, with two pieces of toast topped with banana. Also drink a glass of orange juice.
- Drink at least three glasses of water during the morning: the more fluid in your body the less dehydrated you'll be when you drink alcohol.
- Snack on two pieces of fruit heavy in vitamin C – try kiwi, guava, mango, strawberries or oranges.

Afternoon

- Take another 200mg of milk thistle.
- For lunch, have a grilled chicken breast

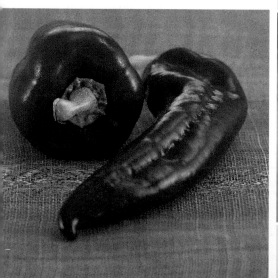

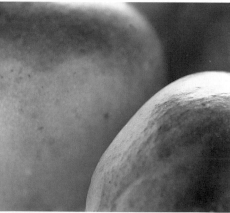

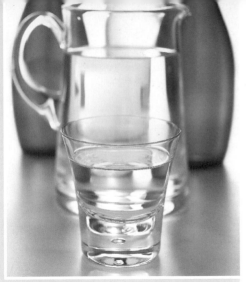

Living the detox life

While the plan should always be used before a big night out, it's also important to drink sensibly the rest of the time. Try following these rules:

- Do not drink more than two units of alcohol on a 'normal' night. A unit consists of: a small glass of wine; 250ml (just under half a pint) of normal-strength beer or a pub measure of spirits. (Remember, strong lagers and large wine glasses can contain up to three units.)
- Drink water with alcohol. Intersperse every drink with a glass or two of water to help replace the fluid you're losing. This speeds the rate at which your body can detox and prevent dehydration.
- If you drink more than three drinks a day, have two to three alcohol-free days afterwards to help your body recover.
- The younger you are the less you should drink. Researchers at the London School of Hygiene & Tropical Medicine in London, UK, have found that alcohol's protective effects are highest in those who start drinking in their 30s. Heavy drinking before then cancels out benefits.
- If you find it hard to cut down, try the herb kudzu (available from health food stores), which is commonly used in China to reduce alcohol cravings. In one UK trial, 64 per cent of volunteers said they were drinking less after taking the herb.
- Know your toxin count. Some drinks are more damaging than others. Generally, the darker the alcohol the more problems it will cause – brandy is the worst. But also beware young wines. Oaked chardonnays and red wines under three years old contain comparatively higher levels of hangover-producing chemicals.

salad; you can make the salad detox-heavy by including spinach, red peppers, tomatoes, artichoke hearts and shredded red cabbage.
- Drink another four glasses of water.
- Snack on two pieces of vitamin-C-rich fruit – or make a smoothie from a glass of milk, two tablespoons of blueberries and two tablespoons of strawberries.

Evening
- Take 1,200mg of N-Acetyl-Cysteine.
- Dine on the perfect mix of protein, carbohydrates and fat. A good meal is spaghetti bolognese: lean mince, red peppers, tomatoes and aubergine served over wholewheat pasta and topped with two tablespoons of grated cheese.
- You can drink one cup of coffee, and you should also try to consume four more glasses of water before the party starts.
- Go out and enjoy yourself.

Before bed
- Take another 200mg of milk thistle.
- Drink 500ml (just under 1 pint) of water, or a large glass of orange juice.

post-party hangover plan

So last night crept up on you, you didn't have time to prepare your body with the Pre-party Plan (see page 74), you overdid it with the alcohol, and this morning you're suffering the inevitable consequences. This is the plan that will help get you back on your feet as soon as physically possible.

About hangovers

To understand how this plan works, you need to understand what a hangover is. The answer to that is toxin poisoning.

All the effects that alcohol has had on your body are ganging up on you and causing painful symptoms. For example, every four alcoholic drinks you drank last night caused up to 1 litre (2 pints) of fluid to be lost from your system. This creates dehydration and causes headaches, fatigue and that parched-mouth feeling. A hangover is also the sign of low blood sugar in the body. Normally, when you sleep, the body fuels itself with glucose stored in the liver; however, when the liver is dealing with alcohol, it stops doing the rest of its jobs. This means that when you wake up your blood-sugar levels are likely to be extremely low, which adds to your fatigue, leaves you feeling sick and light-headed, but also causes those shakes you're trying to hide. Finally, alcohol inflames the lining of your stomach, creating that queasy feeling. That's the bad news; the good news is that, although you can't stop all these symptoms in the next 5 minutes, you can dramatically speed up their demise with this plan.

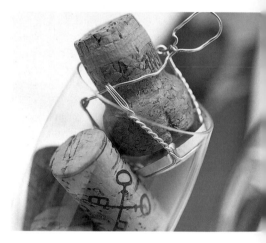

The solution

Natural therapies and exercises can help to ease your body after a heavy night of drinking and can also kick-start it into healing itself.

AROMATHERAPY

Let's start with something that will revive you enough to think about tackling the main part of the programme. When scientists recently looked at the power of lavender oil on the body they found it took just 10 minutes to lower blood pressure; using anti-hangover oils on your body will

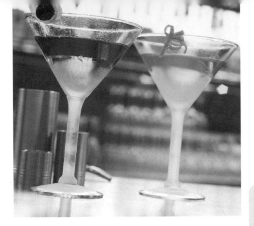

much of the leftover alcohol rushing round your system and only make you feel worse. Instead, just use the following simple posture, called 'Pose of a Child' (see box below), to help gently boost the circulation in your body and promote slow, steady alcohol elimination.

have a similarly rapid effect. The best hangover blend is two drops of fennel oil and two drops of juniper used as an inhalation. Or try some rose oil. The Romans used this oil to fight hangovers because it balances the body, and it doesn't have a diuretic action so won't lead to further dehydration. Add two drops to a carrier oil and massage your hands with the oil, paying particular attention to the fleshy area between your thumb and forefinger. This acupressure point is good at stopping headaches (but don't use in pregnancy).

YOGA

The aromatherapy should have reduced some of your physical symptoms, so it's time to start the body healing itself. A lot of people really swear by exercise to kill a hangover. It works mainly because it releases endorphins that heal the headache, but it also dehydrates you; so, while it can initially help, it can make you feel worse soon afterwards. The same goes for saunas: sweating may eliminate toxins from your system, but they are not good cures for a hangover. Instead, you should try the toxin-releasing effects of yoga. If you only have a mild hangover, try the Simple Yoga Regime (see pages 22–27); however, if you're truly suffering, that's not such a good idea. If you could get through it, it could send too

POSE OF A CHILD

- Sit up on your knees so that your bottom rests on your feet. Breathe in and out slowly and deeply.
- Bend slowly forward from your waist so that your face touches the floor (if you can't reach, put a pillow where your head will land). Turn your face to the left. Relax with your hands hanging alongside your body.
- Keep breathing deeply – this will promote your organs to start detoxing.
- Stay in this position for as long as you feel comfortable.
- Slowly return to your starting position.

Now you're ready to move on to the real plan…

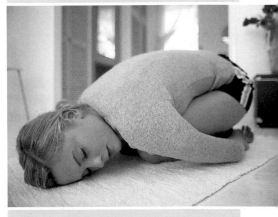

The food solution

What's your natural instinct when you have a hangover? For most of us, it's to reach for food – and that's exactly what you should do.

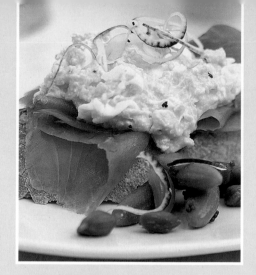

Food is the natural way to detox from a hangover since it provides everything you need to make yourself feel better. First, by eating you help to stabilize your blood-sugar levels. Second, food allows you to replenish the stores of the B vitamins and vitamin C that were destroyed by all that alcohol the night before, thereby recharging your body's natural ability to detox itself.

WHAT TO REACH FOR

Fruit juice. Dehydration is the major cause of most hangover symptoms. Therefore your first defence against them should be trying to boost fluid levels within your body. So why is fruit juice better than water? As well as a good proportion of water, fruit juice also contains antioxidants that help to strengthen the liver. According to research published in a leading toxicology journal, the presence of the fructose in the juice actually helps increase the speed at which the body metabolizes alcohol. Drinking juice and eating fruit throughout the day will also help to replenish lost vitamin C.

Scrambled eggs. Protein is a big hangover helper. To detox properly, your body needs the amino acids found in protein foods. Any will do, but cysteine, which is found in high quantities in eggs, is particularly helpful. Eggs are also good because they contain low levels of fat. Fat is digested through the liver, so is best avoided on hangover mornings or your body switches from detoxing the alcohol to detoxing the fat, leaving you in pain for longer.

Toast and honey. These will help raise blood-sugar levels, taking away that jittery, sick feeling and supplying another dose of detoxing fructose. Brown toast is also high in B vitamins, which need replenishing to boost your energy. Adding other foods rich in B vitamins, such as red meat and wholemeal pasta, throughout the day will maximize these effects.

Leafy green vegetables. Many leafy green vegetables contain natural substances that help support the liver and enable it to work at a faster rate after drinking alcohol. Most of these are not things you want to eat first thing, so spreading them throughout the day can help shorten your hangover without testing your stomach too much. Good ones to try include cruciferous vegetables (like cabbage and broccoli) and artichokes. These vegetables also include levels of folic acid, which is a vital anti-alcohol nutrient because it can actually repair some of the cell damage inflicted by alcohol. Watercress is also good because it contains high levels of chlorophyll, which helps to re-oxygenate the body – and oxygen is something you need lots of as detox can quickly deplete the levels of oxygen in the blood.

Putting the plan into practice

Here's a day-long menu that will help you to eat your way out of that hangover.

First thing

- Drink a glass of orange juice.
- Take up to 200mg of milk thistle with some water. Its effects may not be as effective if you take it after the party rather than before, but it will help support your liver.

Breakfast

- Scrambled eggs and baked beans.
- Brown toast with honey.
- Carrot juice or more orange juice.
- A multivitamin. You should never take vitamins on an empty stomach, so now is the best time to take that vitamin pill.

Mid-morning

- Make a fruit smoothie out of yogurt, blueberries, raspberries and strawberries. Or prepare a fruit salad with orange, kiwi, strawberries and melon.

Lunch

- Chicken or tuna sandwich (on wholemeal bread) with a watercress and tomato salad.
- Carrot, apple or orange juice.
- Another 200mg of milk thistle.

Mid-afternoon

- Toast and honey.

Evening meal

- Lamb chops, with a serving of brown rice, cabbage and artichokes.
- Apple or orange juice.
- A final 200mg of milk thistle.

BEAT THE PAIN NATURALLY

While the day-long diet will help you to detox more quickly, you're probably also wondering if it will also get rid of your headache. It will go eventually, but if you need immediate help, you're going to have to use some other methods.

Your natural instinct is probably to reach for the painkillers, but resist. Paracetamol aggravates the liver, so taking it after drinking alcohol is a very bad idea; aspirin may be kinder on the liver but it upsets the stomach and destroys vitamin C, which is something you need in detox.

Instead, you should try one of the following three natural remedies instead:

White willow bark. This natural painkiller is the ingredient aspirin is made from, but it doesn't irritate your stomach in the same way, nor does it deplete vitamin C levels.

Nux Vom. This homeopathic remedy treats headaches, nausea and constipation.

Breathing exercise. Alcohol decreases the oxygen levels in the body, adding to fatigue and fogged thinking. It is very important that you get more oxygen into your body, as it will help to restore some vitality, so try spending 2 minutes on this simple exercise.

Sit up straight and breathe normally for 30 seconds or so. Now breathe in, expanding rather than contracting your stomach as you do so. Pull the air in so that it fills your lungs, expanding your stomach so that you look pregnant. Hold this position for a second or two, then exhale gently, contracting your lungs and stomach muscles. Repeat the process 5–6 times.

Living the detox life

Simply, don't drink too much alcohol – or at least prepare yourself with the Pre-party Plan (see page 74) next time.

stop smoking plan

Around 70 per cent of all the smokers in the world want to give up the habit, because they know that smoking is bad for their health. If you're reading this, you're probably one of those people – and this plan should make it possible for you to achieve that goal.

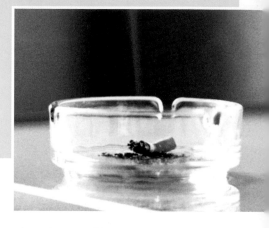

About smoking

According to the UK stop-smoking group ASH, the following benefits result when you give up:

- Twenty minutes after giving up smoking your blood pressure and pulse rate get back to normal.
- Eight hours after your last cigarette nicotine and carbon monoxide levels in the blood reduce by half.
- After 24 hours carbon monoxide is completely eliminated from your body and your lungs start to clear out mucus and other smoking debris.
- Forty-eight hours is all it takes for the nicotine to abate. As your withdrawal symptoms start to diminish your sense of smell and taste will improve.
- Seventy-two hours after your last cigarette you'll find it easier to breathe and you have more energy.
- Over the next 2–12 weeks, the circulation around your whole body begins to improve – you'll notice this most by the glow it gives to your skin.
- Once you've been a non-smoker for three to nine months, your lung function will

have improved by 10 per cent. This helps reduce smokers' symptoms like coughs, wheezing and breathing difficulties. It's also good news for longevity, since people with the best lungs tend to have the longest lives.

- One year after quitting sees your risk of heart attack cut to half that of a smoker.
- When you reach your ten-year milestone your risk of lung cancer will be just half that of a smoker, and in another five years you'll be back to the same risk of heart attack as someone who has never smoked.

All of this happens no matter how old you are, no matter how many cigarettes a day you smoke or how long you've been doing it for. It really is never too late to give up smoking, so why not make today the day you decide to stop?

The solution

The following plan is designed to last about five weeks – the length of time it takes for withdrawal to stop.

There are two main parts: the diet, which you carry out for a fortnight (or more depending on the method you choose to give up); and the controlling cravings plan, which you should carry out for the whole five weeks. But, first, you need to start preparing yourself.

PREPARATION

Getting into the right mind-set to stop smoking is very important. You have to be focused on what you are doing, why you're doing it and how you're doing it. Having all this sorted out will make sticking to the programme much easier. The good news is all this takes just two steps.

Step 1

Decide why you want to quit smoking and write those reasons down – all of them. If you get stuck, think about headings like Health, Looks, Finances, Family, Things I'll be able to do. Now copy these reasons onto another piece of paper headed 'What Will Happen When I've Stopped Smoking', but change the wording of any negative statements into something positive. For example, if you've written 'I won't have to spend money on cigarettes', change that to 'I will have extra money to spend on anything I like'. Or, if one of your reasons is 'I won't cough every morning', change that

to 'My lungs will feel healthier and less congested'. It may sound strange, but, psychologically, positive thinking is usually much more effective than negative. Every morning, read that piece of paper and focus on each of the statements.

Step 2

Now you need to decide how you are going to stop smoking. There are a few methods that you can use, but three work best with the Stop Smoking Plan.

Cold turkey'. This means just stopping without any aids. It's a good approach, but it's also the most intense because you will probably suffer strong nicotine withdrawal for 24–48 hours and milder symptoms for a week to ten days. Using the diet detailed on page 85 will help reduce these, which will make things easier. You should start the diet the day before you decide to stop, then stick to it for at least a fortnight. Also use the controlling cravings tips (see page 87) to help you tackle any urges to smoke that you may develop and keep this up for the next five weeks.

Nicotine replacement therapy (NRT). Nicotine replacement (in the form of patches or gum, for example) supplies a dose of nicotine to the body without you having to ingest smoke. This helps prevent the withdrawal symptoms while you work on stopping the habit of smoking. It's okay to use such a replacement treatment on this detox plan, since nicotine is one of the least harmful ingredients in cigarettes. If you are using NRT, the controlling cravings section is the most important part of the plan for you (see page 87). Use NRT for as long as you need; then, as you start to come off it, you should begin to use the diet to help you beat the withdrawal symptoms that will occur.

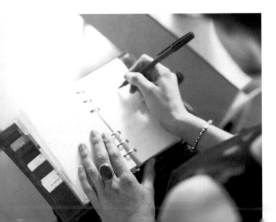

Cutting down. Many experts say this is one of the hardest ways to give up smoking because it just prolongs your addiction. However, if you're afraid of withdrawal, it can give you a safety net. If you're going to use this method, you'll be on the diet for five weeks. While you do this, you should aim to reduce the number of cigarettes you smoke progressively by one-fifth per week. For a 20-a-day smoker, this means either reducing your intake by four cigarettes a day for the whole week (that is, reduce to 16 per day for the first week, 12 per day for the second week, and so on), or cutting down progressively by one cigarette a day on the first four days of the week (that is, 19 on Monday, 18 on Tuesday, 17 on Wednesday, 16 on Thursday, stay at that level for Friday to Sunday, then start reducing again on Monday).

Start with the cigarettes you feel you need most first because if you can break the habit of these, while you have the safety net of being able to smoke if you want one, it's going to be much easier when you get to the last week. Also use the controlling cravings tips to keep you from lighting up when you shouldn't.

Stop smoking diet

All foods have the ability to create within us an acid or an alkaline state, and this acid/alkaline balance is the key to this diet.

When doctors at Columbia University, USA, measured the acidity or alkalinity of smokers' bodies, they found that those with the highest acid balance also smoked the most. The reason for this is that acidity actually increases the speed at which nicotine leaves the body, making you crave another cigarette faster. An alkaline diet, however, slows the rate at which nicotine leaves the system, reducing cravings and making stopping easier. When researchers at the University of Nebraska Medical Centre in the USA tried the diet on smokers cutting down over five weeks, only one was smoking at the end of the trial – and they were only on two cigarettes a day. The others had all stopped.

WHAT ARE ALKALINE FOODS?

All vegetables, particularly watercress, asparagus, alfalfa, courgettes, endive, carrots, potatoes (with the skins on), celery, spinach and swiss chard.

All fruits (except blueberries and cranberries), but especially melon, dates, mango, papaya, kiwi fruit, pineapple, raisins, apricots, avocado and apples.

A selection of other foods, namely tofu, soya milk and cheese, garlic, eggs, almonds, coconuts, natural yogurt, quinoa grain, herb teas and most herbs and spices.

All other foods are acid-forming. Therefore, while you're on the diet, you should aim to eat substantially more alkaline foods in each meal: ideally 70 per cent of your plate should be alkaline foods and 30 per cent acidic. There is an exception: oats (technically an acidic food) have proven to be a powerful weapon against nicotine withdrawal. In research carried out in Ruchill Hospital in Glasgow, UK, smokers given extracts of oats for one month had fewer cravings when they gave up smoking than people on a placebo. It's believed ingredients called alkaloids help calm the body and slow nicotine withdrawal. Plenty of oats are included in the diet, but you can also take a daily supplement or a tincture If you're eating oats at a meal, aim for 50 per cent oats and 50 per cent alkaline food.

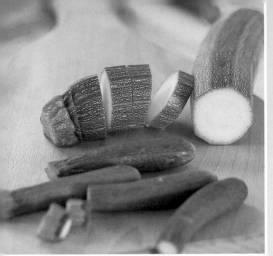

Stop smoking diet

Below, seven days' worth of food are provided to give you some ideas of what you can eat for breakfast, lunch, evening meals and snacks. Mix and match to give yourself a varied diet.

Breakfasts

- Porridge made from oat flakes and soya milk. Top with raisins and serve with two pieces of fruit.
- Fruit plate made from half a mango, a slice of watermelon, slices of pineapple and some dried apricots. Serve with rye bread.
- Baked apple stuffed with raisins. Oatcakes or a small serving of porridge.
- Oatcakes topped with mashed bananas and a handful of strawberries.
- Fruit smoothie made from one banana, two handfuls of raspberries and one glass of orange juice. Serve with rye toast and slices of watermelon.
- Poached egg with grilled tomatoes and mushrooms.
- Oat flapjacks served with a selection of fresh fruit.

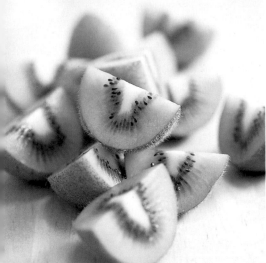

Lunches

- Jacket potato topped with lean protein (such as tuna, ham, cottage cheese, baked beans, chicken, prawns, tofu). Serve this with a large salad of watercress, tomato and red onion.
- Carrot or pumpkin soup served with oatcakes topped with mild cheddar cheese and sliced tomato. Finish with two pieces of fruit.
- Salad consisting of smoked chicken (or cottage cheese) and mango on a bed of lettuce, celery, avocado, cherry tomatoes and alfalfa.

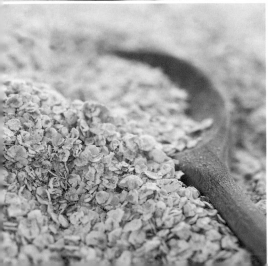

- Open sandwich made up of one slice of rye bread topped with lean protein (see page 85), sliced avocado, sliced tomato and alfalfa. Accompany with a cup of vegetable soup and finish with fruit.
- Salad niçoise made from green beans, tomato, onion and lettuce. Finish this off by topping it with tuna and/or a boiled egg.
- Crudités of carrot, cucumber, celery, cherry tomatoes and pitta bread served with hummus, salsa and guacamole dips. Follow this with a piece of fresh fruit.
- Grilled beefburger or vegetarian burger served with potato salad (keep the potatoes in their skins) and coleslaw.

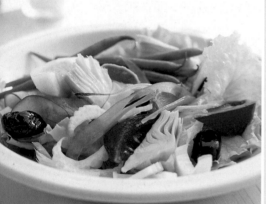

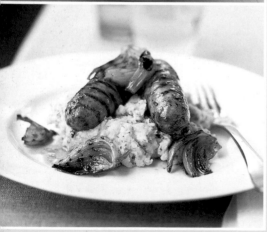

Evening meals

- Vegetable stir-fry with chicken, a little soy sauce and ginger and as many bean sprouts, red peppers, baby corn, mangetout and water chestnuts as you like. Serve on brown rice.
- Lean protein (such as grilled trout, roasted chicken breast, marinated tofu or baked salmon) served with new potatoes and salad of rocket, grilled red peppers and artichoke heart.
- Vegetable curry accompanied by a side serving of dhal and spinach cooked with a little lemon and coriander.
- Low-fat sausages (meat or vegetarian) with mashed potatoes (keep the skins on) and peas.
- Grilled courgettes topped with grated cheese and tomato. Serve this with couscous and mixed grilled vegetables (made from red and yellow peppers, mushrooms and onions).
- Vegetable kebabs served with brown rice. Add a few cubes of cooked chicken, monkfish, king prawns or feta to each kebab if you want to.
- Grilled steak or portabella mushroom served with thick-cut chips (keep the skins on), asparagus spears and watercress and tomato salad.

Snacks

- Fruit.
- A handful of almonds.
- Fruit or vegetable juices or smoothies.
- Crudités served with hummus.
- Oatcakes topped with fruit.

ALLEVIATING SIDE-EFFECTS NATURALLY

When you stop smoking, various side-effects can occur. Here's advice on how to tackle them naturally.

Constipation. Nicotine is a bowel stimulant and without it your system can take up to two weeks to regulate. Take two 5g doses of psyllium husks daily and drink plenty of water.

Coughs. This is just your body clearing out the leftover debris from your cigarettes and they will normally last only one to five days. Drinking plenty of fluids will help speed this up; fenugreek tea also helps thin the mucus, making it less uncomfortable. But don't use this if you're pregnant or trying to get pregnant.

Increased appetite. Sniffing essential oils of fennel (not to be used if you're epileptic or pregnant) or juniper (also not suitable for pregnant women) helps decrease appetite. Camomile tea has a similar effect, but don't use this if you're allergic to ragweed pollen.

Insomnia. One of the best treatments for this is the herb valerian. Take a capsule before going to bed.

Depression. Smoking acts as an anti-depressant in up to 50 per cent of smokers, but the herb St John's wort can help. It can, however, interfere with some medications, so check with your doctor before taking it.

The essential oil of lemon helps increase alkalinity levels in the body. Boost your diet by having a daily massage using 10ml of carrier oil with five drops of lemon, or try a lemon bath with five to six drops added.

CONTROLLING CRAVINGS

While the above diet aims to reduce the strength of nicotine cravings, it's possible they will occur. This is partly because nicotine is incredibly addictive, and so there may be some effects on your body even with the dampening effects of the diet, but there's also a psychological element to cigarette cravings.

Many of us use smoking to tackle emotions. If you're stressed, bored, tired or need to focus, and it has become a natural reaction to reach for a cigarette at these points, when you encounter these feelings as you stop smoking your natural instinct will be to smoke again. But don't give in. Instead, when you feel a craving, if you know why it's happening use the specific craving controller below that suits your true feelings. If you don't know why your craving has been triggered, use the general craving controllers. And remember one thing: according to doctors at the F Hutchinson Cancer Research Centre in Washington, USA, if you can get through the first 24 hours without a cigarette you increase the chance of giving up successfully tenfold. Just focus on one day at a time.

Specific craving controllers

Stress. Many smokers think that cigarettes calm them down, but studies by New York psychiatrist Professor Jeffrey Grant Johnson actually showed the opposite. This doesn't make you feel any better, however, if you're getting wound up but can't reach for a cigarette to help. In this case, inhaling oil of lavender is the fastest way to reduce symptoms. You'll find some other 5-minute fixes on page 71.

To clear your head. If you used to smoke in order to help you think, try sniffing peppermint oil or, if you prefer, drinking peppermint tea instead. Studies at the University of Cincinnati, USA, found this helped people think more clearly; in fact, testers scored 28 per cent higher on accuracy tests when using it.

Needing something to do with your hands. This is quite simple – do something else. Doodle, play computer games, squeeze stress balls – anything that keeps your hands occupied.

Low energy. If you're used to smoking to lift your energy when your blood-sugar levels get low, you'll need to prevent this. Try eating little and often, or snack on fruit as that will give your energy a rapid lift without a subsequent fall. The ideal smoker's snack is a satsuma. This is because the segments will help feed the hand-to-mouth action you're used to, while the citrus scent energizes the mind. Ginger tea and the supplement ginseng can also provide a fast lift.

Smoking chair. If you find yourself wanting to smoke in a particular chair or when you watch a particular TV programme, try inhaling some frankincense oil at this point.

This is used to help break ties with the past: the Bach flower remedy Honeysuckle has similar effects.

General craving controllers

Black pepper oil. Add three drops to a tissue and inhale if you feel a craving coming on. Studies in the *Journal of Drug and Alcohol Dependence* showed that it cut nicotine cravings, possibly because it causes the same feeling in the back of the throat.

Nicotiana. This essence from the family of American Flower Essences is made from the leaves of a flowering tobacco plant. Take a few drops on your tongue each day to reduce cravings, or use it when one hits.

Lobelia. This herb has actions similar to those of nicotine in the body, and can therefore be used if your cravings are very bad. It is, however, an incredibly powerful herb and therefore you should never use it without being under the strict supervision of a herbalist.

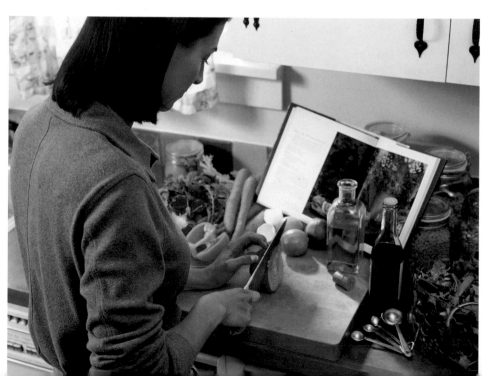

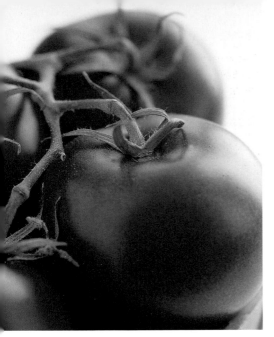

Curled tongue breaths. This yoga technique is said to reduce tobacco cravings possibly because it mimics the action of smoking. To do this, sit upright and breathe normally. Now stick your tongue out and curl it up at the sides to form a tube. Next, inhale slowly through the tube. Put your tongue in and breathe normally for a few seconds. Then repeat the whole process for as long as the craving lasts. (If you find you can't roll your tongue, go back to using one of the other general controllers.)

'If your reaction has been to smoke when you feel bored, stressed or tired, then as you stop your instinct will be to smoke when you encounter these emotions again. But don't give in.'

Living the detox life

Once you've successfully stopped smoking, staying away from cigarettes is the main way to lead the detox life; however, you can also take some steps to help repair some of the damage smoking has caused in your body.

- **Start taking multivitamins.** A host of nutrients can help repair some of the damage that will have occurred in the body. Vitamin B12, for example, can help rebuild cells in the lungs, and vitamin B3 opens up cells that nicotine has damaged. You should not take individual supplements, however, since this can imbalance the body and has been shown to be dangerous in smokers; instead protect yourself by regularly taking a good multivitamin.
- **Eat at least three tomato-based meals a week.** The antioxidant nutrient lycopene found in tomatoes seems to offer protection against the damage caused by smoking.
- **Start drinking green tea.** Japanese researchers found less cell damage in smokers who drank green tea, and it's possible that the tea may help mop up damage after smoking.
- **Avoid passive smoking.** A night spent in a room full of heavy smokers is the same as smoking four cigarettes yourself – so why re-do old damage? If you can't avoid smoky places, at least do the next best thing and increase your consumption of orange juice and watercress; both of these have been shown to speed the rate at which the body excretes the harmful byproducts of smoking.

energizing plan

If there are some mornings when you can't summon up the energy to get up and go, or you just feel tired and lethargic all the time, then this is the plan for you. In as few as three days, you can reinvigorate your body, improve your energy levels and bring back that lost enthusiasm for life.

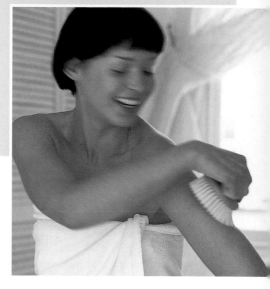

About energy and toxins

Energy is created in the body from food. When we eat, our bodies break down the ingested food into glucose, which is the main sugar that we use for fuel.

It can do this from any food: doughnuts, rare steaks, plates of spinach topped with lemon juice. Healthy or unhealthy, the body can use food as energy. However, its favourite sources are carbohydrate foods like fruit, vegetables, bread, pasta and rice, because these are easy to convert. When the food has been broken down, it is combined with oxygen. This 'burns' the sugar and turns it into a unit of energy called adenosine triphosphate, which the cells then store and use as they need it. In a healthy, fatigue-free body, this process works with no problems and, as a result, we spend each day fully functioning and raring to go. But if the energy process breaks down this is when we start to feel tired.

SO WHAT GOES WRONG?

There are a huge number of things that can interfere with the energy process, but what follows are details of the four main reasons.

You don't have enough nutrients to trigger energy conversion. Like everything in the body, energy production is powered by vitamins, primarily the eight B vitamins and the antioxidant Q10. Also vital are minerals – particularly calcium, magnesium, iron, chromium and zinc. Lack of nutrients can occur because you don't eat the right foods, or because toxins like alcohol or stress destroy them.

You don't have enough blood sugar to produce energy quickly and cleanly. Some carbohydrates are too effective at creating glucose in the body. Refined carbohydrates such as white bread, rice and pasta, or sugary foods like biscuits and cakes, create sudden peaks of glucose in the blood. If large quantities of these are eaten the body panics and, instead of using the glucose for fuel, it hides it in the liver or in fat. Next time cells need energy they have to pull

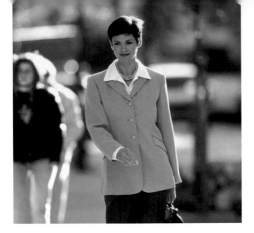

'Sometimes the energy process breaks down, and this is when we start to feel tired.'

The solution

What follows is written as a daily plan, but to get noticeable results you should follow the plan for at least three consecutive days. Doing this will double your energy levels over the course of a long weekend. However, one week is the optimum time to follow the programme for the best results.

stored glucose out of the liver, which fatigues the body.

You don't have enough oxygen in the system. Without oxygen, the body can't burn glucose. Many of us are deprived of oxygen because we breathe so shallowly, but oxygen deprivation can also occur through poor circulation or if our red blood cells (which are the part of blood that carry oxygen) aren't in perfect shape.

You don't have enough mitochondria. Mitochondria are the constituents of cells that turn glucose into fuel. If the levels of these are low, they can't perform as well and toxins, particularly those found in pesticides, actually destroy mitochondria.

What the Energizing Plan aims to do is counteract all these problems. For best results, you should carry out the Lighten-up Plan (see page 44) for at least three days before you start the Energizing Plan. This will remove any immediate toxins hanging around the system, allowing your body to respond more effectively to the energy boost. If that's not possible, at least skip alcohol and excess sugar while you're on this plan. If you're under stress, it would be a good idea to use some of the 5-minute fixes (see page 71) to help relax you, because stress saps energy.

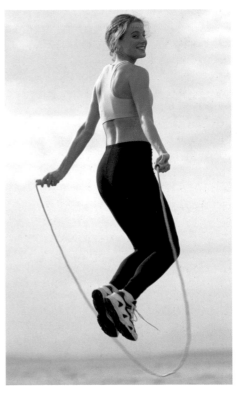

The energizing routine

This may seem like a complicated plan, but it's actually quite simple to follow

7.22am Time to wake up – in an energy-boosting world you shouldn't get up before 7.22am. According to research carried out by the University of Westminster, London, UK, doing so creates higher than normal levels of the energy-sapping hormone cortisol in your body. Researchers found that people with high levels of cortisol tend to feel more hassled and fatigued throughout the day. If work pressures mean 7.22am is a lie-in, then at least wake your body more gently by using a daylight alarm clock (check health magazines for advertisements). These slowly raise the levels of light in the room, waking you slowly and calmly.

7.30am Take one multivitamin supplement, one probiotic supplement and one capsule of fish oil (or if you are vegetarian one of evening primrose oil) with a large glass of water. This is the first of

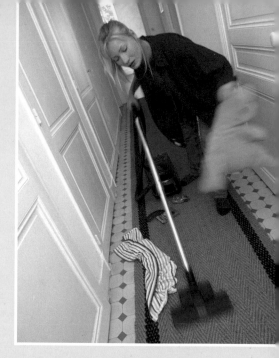

eight glasses you'll drink over the day – aim for one an hour. The supplements will provide energy and nutrients and aid your digestion, maximizing the nutrients you absorb from food. Leave half an hour between taking these and eating.

7.40am Carry out the 'Salute to the Sun' exercise (see page 69). This yoga programme is stimulating and energizing and will help prepare you for the day ahead. It takes about 5 minutes, and should be done outside or at least facing a window, which adds to your energy banks because sunlight stops production of the sleep-inducing hormone melatonin.

7.50am Body-brush (see page 28). This will stimulate your circulation, helping increase levels of oxygen flooding the system. Finish with a shower. Chinese therapists believe that as well as freshening you up, running water helps wash away negative vibrations.

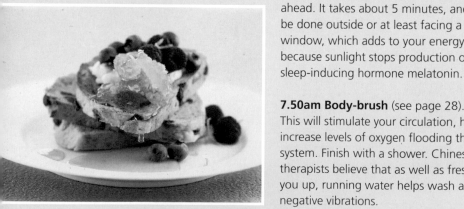

8am Get your breakfast B vitamins.
B vitamins are vital to the energy levels of your body, and breakfast foods provide excellent levels of them. For best results, choose a bowl of bran cereal with skimmed milk, and two pieces of wholewheat toast with a little honey and some fruit. If you normally have coffee in the morning, have

Oxygen Juice

6 slices of pineapple (fresh or tinned) • 1 banana • 6 fresh strawberries • 1 handful of wheatgrass
Put each item through the juicer, then mix together and shake well.

Suggested lunch menu

- Start with a glass of Oxygen Juice.
- Now choose from one of the following energizing vegetable bases, using as much of each vegetable as you like.
  Fluid Fuel: lettuce, cucumber, celery, chopped apple and a few slices of pear.
  Quick Cleanse: asparagus, cherry tomatoes and yellow peppers on a bed of alfalfa.
  Steamed and Simple: steamed green cabbage, carrot, mushrooms, asparagus and mangetout.
  Sunshine Salad: watercress, carrot, beetroot and pink grapefruit.
- Add a 50g (2oz) portion of one (or a mix) of the following: salmon, anchovies, mackerel, herring, trout, sardines, sunflower, pumpkin or sesame seeds, walnuts or cashews, tahini. These protein foods create a slowly burned form of energy that your body can use throughout the afternoon, but also provide high levels of essential fatty acids, which the red blood cells need to travel through the body. If you're vegetarian, it can be hard to get enough essential fatty acids, so adding two teaspoons of flaxseed oil to your salad may help boost levels.

it; research from the University of Bristol, UK, reveals that if you're used to having a morning cuppa – tea or coffee – skipping it will leave you more tired.

10am 'De-junk' your day. Energy isn't just sapped physically from our bodies, it's also sapped mentally by stress, worry and feelings of being overwhelmed. Whether you work in an office or are busy at home, clearing physical and mental clutter should be your first job. Tidy your desk, put away the kids' toys or first tackle the one task you really don't want to do. When this is finished, it will feel like a weight has been lifted and your energy will start to soar.

11am Time for a snack. Not only does eating little and often keep the blood-sugar levels of the body stable, but it also boosts energy in other ways. Digesting foods uses energy in the body (in fact 10 per cent of

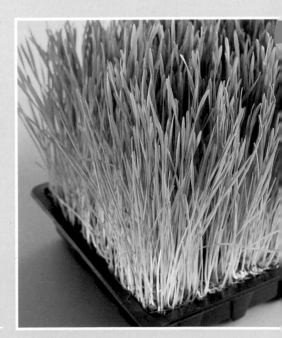

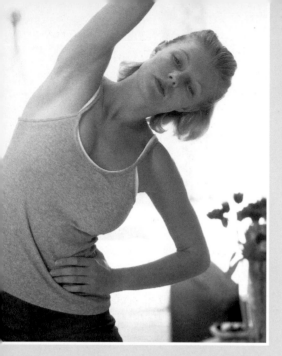

(along with alfalfa) helps neutralize the natural toxin ammonia produced within your body, which is an extremely common cause of fatigue.

3pm Head outside. By now, the air in your office, or even at home, is likely to be low in oxygen, boosting your feelings of fatigue. Five minutes of fresh air now can stimulate you to finish the day, so go for a quick walk. If that's not possible, try the following yoga technique called 'Bellows Breath', which oxygenates the entire body.

Stand up straight and clench your fists. Breathe in quickly through your nose and out through your mouth. As you do this, pump your arms to get blood circulating around your body. Repeat this process for 1 minute, but listen to your body as you do this. The sudden flood of oxygen can make you feel light-headed and, if this happens, you should stop and breathe normally for a while. It's also good to have some more fruit at this time.

the calories the body uses throughout the day are used in digestion), and meals that are too large can actually fatigue the body. Snacks take the edge off your appetite and stop you over-eating at main meals. A good snack would be two or three citrus fruits; ingredients called flavonoids within these have been shown to thin the blood, which helps to prevent red blood cells clumping together and maximizes oxygen flow.

1pm Eat a good lunch. This meal should be used to boost oxygen and fluid levels in the body, giving you energy to face the afternoon when energy levels naturally dip. Oxygen-boosting foods are those that contain chlorophyll, which has been shown to help rebuild red blood cells. Try wheatgrass, watercress, spinach, dark cabbage, lettuce, alfalfa and other sprouts. You'll also want to fill up on fluid-heavy foods like celery, cucumber, fennel, apples, pears, watermelon, grapefruit and grapes. Finally, include some asparagus, since this

6pm Do some exercise. Toxins have the ability to sap our energy by acting negatively on the mitochondria within the body. However, if you build muscle through exercise you also build mitochondria. Take 30 minutes every other day on the plan to do some kind of aerobic or resistance training, and ideally do it between 4pm and 7pm. Studies at Liverpool John Moores University, UK, have shown that exercise feels easiest at this time of day.

8pm Eat your evening meal. Overnight the body regenerates and naturally detoxes, so the focus of your evening meal should be to provide detoxing foods to boost this process. You should combine these with carbohydrates; while these are primarily energy-givers, in doses of more than 75g (3oz) at one time they can calm the body, which will help boost sleep.

9pm Blend yourself a bedtime bath.
Getting a good night's sleep is vital to boosting energy: it's how the body recharges. It's been shown that bathing aids the sleep process by stimulating the natural cooling process the body uses to trigger sleep hormones. You'll add to sleep effects if you place some essential oils in your bath. One of the best to use here is marjoram. It's very sedative, but also fortifying to the body, which will help you create strength for the next day. Add three drops of marjoram and three drops of calming mandarin to your bath, sit back and relax. If you're pregnant, don't use the marjoram, but stick with the mandarin.

Suggested evening meal menu
- Start with a cup or glass of Winter Warmer Soup (see page 46).
- Choose one of these four bases, using as much of each vegetable as you like.
  Detox Salad: watercress, celery, cucumber, cherry tomato, artichoke hearts.
  Cleansing Coleslaw: white cabbage, onion, grated carrot, sliced beetroot.
  Roast Energy: grill or oven-bake slices of red pepper, yellow pepper, aubergine, onion and mushrooms until soft.
  Steamed and Simple: steamed carrot, mangetout, cauliflower, spinach, asparagus.
- Add a 75g (3oz) serving of one (or a mix) of the following to your chosen base: brown rice, jacket potato, new potatoes, mashed potatoes, wholewheat pasta, couscous, mashed swede, roast parsnips, corn on the cob, sweetcorn, rye, pumpernickel or wholegrain bread.

Living the detox life
Most of what you need to live the detox life is included within the Energizing Plan: add plenty of B vitamins to your diet; boost oxygen intake by breathing and stretching the body regularly; expend energy through exercise to boost energy in the body and, very importantly, get a good night's sleep.

If you can do all those things, you will probably never suffer from fatigue again. However, there's one final thing you can do to help things: read and follow the advice in the 'Living the detox life' section of the Anti-pollution Plan (see page 55). Increasingly, experts believe that a build-up of serious toxins (like the residues of pesticides or heavy metals) in the body is the cause of problems such as chronic fatigue syndrome. Reducing your intake of these is therefore another step in living an energized life.

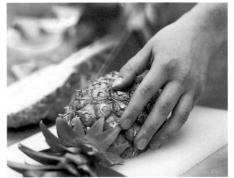

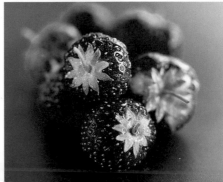

good health plan

This is the plan to use if you feel an illness coming on, or just before the cold and flu season in order to strengthen your body against the possibility of infection. It's also the plan for you if you suffer from niggling health problems such as migraine, arthritis or allergies.

About health and toxins

While this whole book is about improving health and body function, this plan tackles what most of us think of as 'health' – the ability to fight off germs and prevent other problems.

The ability to do this depends on having a strong, balanced immune system. The immune system has a number of elements. First are physical barriers like the skin, the tiny hairs within the nose and lungs (called cilia) and the lining of the stomach and bowel, all of which prevent bacterial entry to the body. Plus, the body has a second wave of defence: the white blood cells, which attack invading bacteria. These cells travel in the blood and lymphatic systems. If these systems are inhibited so is the immune system, and we succumb to germs.

Our immune systems break down for a number of reasons, and experts believe that toxins play a part. It's been shown that alcohol lowers the numbers of a white blood cell called a lymphocyte, making us more susceptible to infection. Similarly, our ability to fight infection is lowered for four hours after a hefty dose of sugar. Stress is different. At first, it boosts the immune system, but if prolonged it depresses immunity and resistance to infection.

Toxic overload can damage our barrier systems: cigarette smoke damages the cilia,

for example. The good news is that caffeine doesn't seem to have any effect either way.

So, it's clear that reducing alcohol, sugar and stress in the run-up to a cold season is a good thing. The Good Health Plan shows you a number of positive ways to improve your immune system, which will help you stop catching every cough and cold around.

IMMUNE-SYSTEM PROBLEMS

The most common problem our immune system faces is invading germs, but there are others. An over-active immune system begins to attack substances that are, to most people, harmless – this happens with allergies. Instead of ignoring house dust or pollen, the body registers it as an invader and attacks it, creating classic symptoms. A more serious problem are auto-immune diseases, in which the body mistakes its own cells for invaders and attacks them. A common example is rheumatoid arthritis, where white blood cells attack joint tissues, creating pain and inflammation.

The solution

If you do everything in the plan for two to three weeks prior to the onset of the cold and flu season (and during the event itself) it should help fight off ailments and ills effectively.

Top 10 immune boosters

Below you will find ten ways to help boost your immune system. These methods can be used in two ways. Either use one, two (or more) of them to help boost your immune system if you feel yourself coming down with a cold or other illness or take them in advance as detailed above.

1 INCREASE VITAMIN C INTAKE

This increases white blood cell numbers by up to ten times in some cases, and also helps boost excretion of a chemical called interferon that prevents viruses from multiplying. The body can store up to 3g of vitamin C a day, and to aid immunity this is the recommended dose. Therefore take a 1g supplement three times daily. Also boost your intake of citrus fruits, red peppers, blueberries and other fruits and vegetables that are rich in vitamin C – ingredients called bioflavonoids in many of these enhance vitamin C performance.

2 BALANCE THE REST OF YOUR DIET

While vitamin C is vital, a truly strong immune system also needs high levels of B vitamins, beta-carotene, vitamin D, calcium, magnesium, iron and zinc. Aim for a good mix of wholegrain carbohydrates, lean proteins and lots of green vegetables to deliver these every day in the cold season, and take a multivitamin for insurance too.

3 TAKE ECHINACEA

This pretty pink flower is a potent immune booster. Scientists at Germany's University of Leipzig found that numbers of macrophage cells (ones that eat bacteria) doubled after they gave patients 30 drops of echinacea tincture three times a day for five days. Unlike multivitamins, echinacea shouldn't be taken every day; instead, use it for one week a month during the cold season, or for five to seven days if you find yourself getting cold symptoms at any other time of year. When using it this way, take 20–30 drops twice a day.

4 EXERCISE

Stimulating the lymphatic system and increasing the numbers of disease-fighting cells in the body are the ways in which exercise helps fight illness; however, if you do too much, exercise actually depresses immunity. Stick to burning 1,200–1,800 calories a week to get the perfect mix of fitness and health benefits.

5 THINK HAPPY THOUGHTS

Viruses enter cells through little holes (called receptors) in the cell's surface. Chemicals produced when we are excited about something, or happy, actually block these holes. Negative emotions, on the other hand, make it easier for bugs to take hold. Studies found that stressed people had 15 per cent more chance of catching a cold when exposed to the virus than people who were more relaxed.

6 GET ENOUGH SLEEP

When the immune system is working to fight illness we get sleepy; it is thought that the body tries to make us conserve energy to fight the bacteria. However, the reverse is also true: when we sleep, the immune system gets more active. If you're not getting the right amount of sleep for your body, it can't fight germs as effectively. Minimize late nights during the cold and flu season, or if you feel a bug coming on.

(7) GET SUNLIGHT

While sunburn is bad for us, some sunlight is good. Russian research has shown that exposure to ultraviolet rays doubles the ability of white blood cells to destroy bacteria. As well as this, sunlight provides our body with vitamin D, which it needs for immunity. Aim to get at least 30 minutes of sunlight or, failing that, natural daylight each day.

(8) STIMULATE YOUR LYMPHATIC SYSTEM

Good circulatory and lymphatic systems are vital to help the body fight infection fast: if they are sluggish, disease-fighting cells can't move effectively around the body. You can boost lymph flow by body-brushing daily, by massage or by using the yoga regime on pages 22–27. However, the simplest way to boost lymph flow is to stimulate what natural therapists call the lymph pump in the sole of the foot. To do this, spend 2–3 minutes a day rising up on your toes and contracting your calf muscles.

(9) WASH YOUR HANDS REGULARLY

Most germs enter the body through the nose or eyes when we touch our face. Washing your hands hourly cuts the amount of germs on them, and so reduces the risk of infection. When US Navy recruits in Illinois, USA, did this, they cut their sick days by 45 per cent.

(10) GET HOT AND SWEATY

Our immune systems work better at a slightly higher temperature than normal body temperature. It's possible that a sauna helps increase immunity, albeit only temporarily. It's a good idea, therefore, to have one once every two to three days.

DETOX SOLUTIONS FOR SPECIFIC HEALTH PROBLEMS

For some people, health problems aren't things that just come and go, and they don't necessarily involve bugs and germs. If you suffer from problems such as migraines, pre-menstrual syndrome, nasal allergies, arthritis or the digestive disorder irritable bowel syndrome, health problems can be a part of daily (or at least monthly) life. However, increasingly, research shows that detoxing can help these conditions. In such cases, you're not necessarily reducing your intake of traditional toxins or avoiding things like air pollution (although this will make a difference). Instead, you should be tackling specific toxins that worsen your problem; these can be something as traditionally healthy as citrus fruits or tomatoes. By cutting these out of your diet, you could therefore reduce symptoms of your problem: this is called an elimination diet.

To carry out a simple elimination diet, you should cut out all the foods linked to your problem for two weeks. Then, one by one, introduce a food for two to three days, eating fairly high quantities of that food during this period; if you don't get any symptoms during that time then that product doesn't cause a problem for you and you can start eating it again. If you do get symptoms, then that is a trigger food and it is best avoided. If you still get symptoms when all linked foods have been eliminated, food may not be the cause of your problem, or you may be sensitive to another food or toxin and you'll need expert help. Just one word of warning: while it's fine to do this for hayfever and nasal allergies, as described below, don't try it without supervision for any food allergies or if you also get asthma with your problem. If you want help in these cases, ask your doctor for a supervised elimination diet.

Migraines

Common triggers: Red wine, cheese, chocolate, eggs, citrus fruit, wheat, tea, coffee, corn, peas and bananas.

What may help: Eat at regular times and increase your levels of magnesium, calcium and fibre (found in leafy green vegetables) – high levels of these may help. Feverfew also helps – research at Nottingham University, UK, found migraines reduced by 24 per cent in people taking a daily dose of 250mg.

Rheumatoid arthritis

Common triggers: Dairy products, citrus fruit, corn, wheat, potatoes, tomatoes, nuts and coffee.

What may help: Both red and white wine help fight the inflammation that causes rheumatoid arthritis; the recommended dose according to researchers at the University of Pisa, Italy is two glasses a day. Evening primrose or starflower oils also help. Aim for enough supplements to provide you daily with 1.4g of gamma linolenic acid (GLA), which is the active ingredient in the oils (check packets for the dosage).

Irritable bowel syndrome

Common triggers: Fatty foods, corn, tea, coffee, wheat, dairy products and citrus fruit.

What may help: Peppermint oil is one of the commonest, safest treatments for irritable bowel syndrome (IBS). In trials at Hope Hospital in Manchester, UK 80 per cent of patients taking peppermint oil found their IBS symptoms improved. The recommended dose is 0.2–0.4ml, given in capsule form only, three times daily.

Pre-menstrual syndrome

Common triggers: Coffee, tea, sugar, alcohol, salt and chocolate.

What may help: Eating high-carbohydrate foods little and often. This balances blood-sugar levels and helps reduce the mood swings and food cravings that can be linked to pre-menstrual syndrome (PMS). High levels of magnesium and calcium (in leafy green vegetables) can also help. The herb agnus castus has also been shown to have benefits with PMS, because it helps balance hormones. German researchers giving their patients 40 drops of liquid agnus castus daily for five months found that 90 per cent of their patients stopped getting PMS.

Hayfever and rhinitis

Common triggers: Melon, plums, apples, tomatoes, celery and carrots.

What may help: Onions, citrus fruit, tea and garlic. These contain the antioxidant quercetin, which Japanese research has shown causes cells to release less histamine. Other dietary factors that have been shown to help reduce allergy symptoms are oily fish (try for two to three portions a week) and increasing dietary levels of magnesium.

Living the detox life

If you want to keep your immunity boosted all year, just integrate the ten tips given earlier into your everyday life.

The exception to this is echinacea, which can lose efficacy if used too often. Keep that for the cold season. For the specific health problems described above, once the food has been eliminated from the diet for a few months, most people can eat small quantities every so often. If it turned out that a favourite food was the cause, try one to two portions a week and monitor your symptoms. If they return, try one or two more but don't overdo it. Remember it's over-exposure that leads to intolerance.

weight-loss plan

If you want to lose weight but have found that diets never work, this is the plan for you. It explains why toxic exposure can slow even the most devoted weight-watching plans, and teaches you how to beat this problem and finally get down to your desired size and shape.

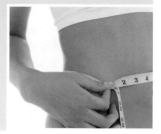

About weight and toxins

In the eyes of most of us there are only two types of weight problem: you're gaining it too fast or you're losing it too slowly. According to traditional dieticians both of these have their root in the same cause: the number of calories you are taking in is more than the number you are using up. Basically this is true, but it doesn't mean that certain factors, like toxins, can't interfere too.

FAT GAIN

Most of us know that what we eat determines whether or not we get fat, but new research is revealing that there's more to this reaction than how many calories are in a dish. In her book, *The Detox Diet*, Paula Baillie Hamilton (Penguin, 2002) explains that many of the foods we eat now contain toxins that actually promote weight gain in animals, and are likely to do this in humans too. To make matters worse, because many of these toxins appear in pesticides, they are concentrated in foods that we would use to lose weight, such as salad crops, soft fruits and other fruits and vegetables; even if you eat organic, you can be exposed to these toxins from insecticides and other household products.

FAT-BURNING INHIBITORS

It's not just major toxins that cause problems with weight gain. Relatively harmless toxins like caffeine or alcohol also play a role, because they destroy the vital nutrients we need to burn fat. Recent research from the University of Tennessee, USA, found that the more calcium there was in a diet the more fat the body burned, since calcium has the power to convert cells from fat storers into fat burners. Caffeine, however, actually causes us to excrete calcium, taking out 6mg from our stores with every cup of coffee we drink.

Free radicals produced when toxins enter the body, or are processed, can also remove vital fat-burning nutrients. Research published in the *European Journal of Clinical Nutrition* showed that 58 per cent of overweight women were deficient in vitamin C (one of the major free radical fighting antioxidants); and in trials where overweight women were given vitamin C supplements they lost weight even without dieting. Deficiencies in another antioxidant, vitamin E, are also linked to excess weight, and this could be linked to toxic overload.

Magnesium is important for fat-burning, and it is destroyed by stress – a toxin that causes problems in other ways since it increases levels of a hormone called cortisol. Not only does cortisol stimulate your appetite, but it also encourages fat cells in the abdominal area to store fat.

FLUID RETENTION

Toxins can also interfere with your ability to lose weight because you have gained fluid. Unprocessed toxins are stored in the fat if the liver can't handle them; stored with them, however, are large amounts of water. The reason for this is that the body's 'solution to pollution is dilution'. This means that if the body thinks something is harmful it will surround it with water to minimize its strength and efficacy. If you're storing high levels of toxins, you're also probably carrying lots of fluid. If so, no amount of fat-burning will reduce your weight.

In some people, this reaction occurs for another reason: food intolerance. This arises when the body loses the ability to digest a particular type of food properly. Food stays in the system longer than it should and it ferments, filling the body with substances that it finds toxic.

The solution

This mixes diet, exercise and massage to tackle the toxic causes of weight gain.

It is recommended that you stick to the plan for a month, after which you will have lost up to 6.5kg (1 stone), depending on how much fluid you retain. After a month, if you still have more to lose, follow the advice in 'Extending the plan'. If you don't, go straight to 'Living the detox life'.

If you follow the advice given in the 'Living the detox life' section of the Anti-pollution Plan (see page 55) before you start, you can enhance the plan's effects.

Weight-loss diet

This is the main part of the Weight-loss Plan. Even the most devoted fitness experts admit that when you're trying to lose weight 80 per cent of the results come from a healthy diet.

However, rather than just cutting calories, this diet also aims to reduce the amount of fluid in your body by introducing foods that prevent fluid retention (bananas, prunes, orange juice and dried apricots), and by cutting out wheat and dairy-based foods, which are the ones most commonly linked to food intolerances. The diet is also low in sodium, which will also reduce the amount of fluid you retain. In addition, it supplies large amounts of detox foods and supplements that will help neutralize any harmful toxins released into the body as the fat breaks down. This is important, so please don't skip your daily Antioxidant Cocktail (see page 101). It will also boost your efforts if you use organic products and keep toxins such as alcohol to a minimum so that your liver can deal with any released toxins.

You shouldn't get hungry on this diet, as you are eating regularly; but, if you do, don't give in to the craving. While detoxing enhances results, it's cutting calories that ensures weight comes off, so try acupressure instead. The appetite point is on your ear about 1cm (½in) from the top; on the side next to your head you'll feel a small hollow. Use a cotton bud to press it gently a few times.

Early morning

- Take a multivitamin and mineral supplement plus 1g of vitamin C.
- Take 2,000mg of conjugated linoleic acid (CLA). In Swedish research,

patients taking this healthy fat for 14 weeks lost 3.8 per cent of their body fat, even when they didn't change their diet.
- Take 5g of psyllium.
- Wash these down with two glasses of water, and aim to drink at least eight more during the day.

Breakfast (eat this half an hour after your supplements)
- Start with a glass of Antioxidant Cocktail.
- Choose a high-fibre breakfast from the list below. Fibre not only fills you up, but it also reduces the number of calories you absorb from food. Wholegrain cereals also contain antioxidants and have the ability to bind to some toxins in the bowel.
  Bowl of bran cereal topped with soya milk and a handful of prunes.
  One cored apple filled with raisins and baked in a preheated oven for 30 minutes at 220°C (425°F) or Gas Mark 7. Top this with soya yogurt.
  Two slices of rye or pumpernickel toast spread with honey. One boiled egg.
  Porridge made from oat flakes and water or soya milk. Mix in a handful of chopped dried apricots.
  Two oatcakes topped with mashed banana and strawberries.

Mid-morning snack
- Two pieces of fruit and a cup of dandelion tea. Dandelion helps the body excrete excess fluid without destroying other vital nutrients.

Lunchtime
- Half an hour before lunch, take another 1,000mg of CLA and 5g of psyllium and wash these down with at least two glasses of water.

Antioxidant Cocktail
50g (2oz) prepared blueberries • 50g (2oz) prepared strawberries • ½ mango • 250ml (8floz) orange juice
Put all the ingredients into a blender and blend until smooth.

Supercleanse Soup
1 small onion, finely chopped • 1.5 litres (2½ pints) light chicken stock or water • 2 small potatoes, diced • 2 large handfuls of spinach • 1 large bunch of watercress, stems removed • salt and pepper
Cook the onion in 2–3 tablespoons of chicken stock or water for 1 minute. Add the potatoes, seasoning and the rest of the stock/water. Bring to the boil and simmer until the potatoes are soft. Add the spinach and watercress and stir for 3 minutes. Remove from the heat and blend in a liquidizer. This recipe will make enough soup for a couple of days so you can store it in the fridge and have some another day.

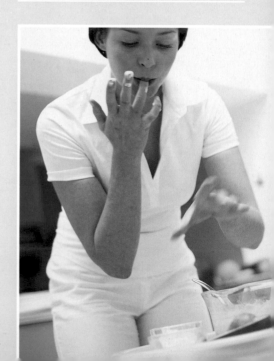

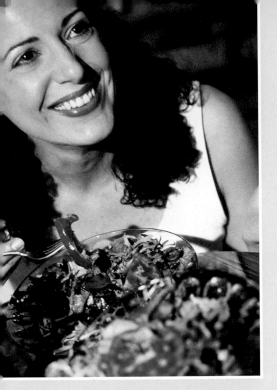

Stir-fry Sensation: in a tiny amount of oil that has sliced ginger in it, stir-fry the following vegetables – asparagus spears, bean sprouts, shredded green cabbage, mangetout and broccoli.

Good-for-you Grill: grill mushrooms, thinly sliced aubergine, red onions, yellow peppers and courgettes until they soften.

- Then drizzle each base with any of the following: balsamic vinegar, 1 teaspoon of olive oil containing some chopped chilli (chilli boosts the metabolism), a spoonful of salsa, lemon juice or fat-free vinaigrette. Top with 75g (3oz) of lean protein such as chicken, turkey, salmon, tuna, mackerel, sardines, anchovies, lean ham, lean roast beef, a bean blend made up of kidney beans, green beans and chickpeas or grilled or marinated tofu.

Afternoon snack

- Two more pieces of fruit.

Evening meal

- Start with another 1,000mg of CLA, plus a glass of Chelating Cocktail (see page 53) or, if you prefer, a bowl of the Supercleanse Soup.
- Choose one of the vegetable bases from the lunch options, but this time top it with 50g (2oz) of lean protein and 50g (2oz) of carbohydrates such as a jacket potato, new potatoes, mashed potatoes, roast sweet potatoes, rye or pumpernickel bread, mashed swede, parsnips or pumpkin, sweetcorn or corn-on-the-cob, brown rice or wheat-free pasta.

Before bed

- Slice of rye or pumpernickel bread topped with half a banana or a teaspoonful of honey, whichever you prefer.

- As explained in the Anti-pollution eating Plan (see page 52), chelating foods are those that are able to bind to dangerous pollutants in the body, which helps to detox them from the body. Lunch focuses on high quantities of these foods in order to help reduce toxin levels in the body.
- Start with a glass of Chelating Cocktail (see page 53).
- Now choose from one of the following vegetable bases, using as much of each vegetable as you like, except for avocado, which you should limit to half a fruit due to its high calorie content.

Spicy Salad: alfalfa sprouts, tomato, red pepper, black olives, radish.

Clarifying Coleslaw: shredded white cabbage, grated carrot, sliced beetroot, sliced onion.

Pure Power: watercress, cucumber, tomato, artichoke hearts and avocado.

Weight-loss exercise programme

The point of this programme is to help you burn fat, but also to detox the system by stimulating the lymph flow and blood circulation. As a result, you will be combining aerobic exercise with a fat-burning and detox yoga programme (see right). For each week you are on the weight-loss diet, carry out the following.

Monday: 30–60 minutes of aerobic exercise (you can break this up into 10-minute bursts if it makes life easier).

Tuesday: 20–30 minutes of brisk walking, plus the fat-burning and detox yoga programme.

Wednesday: 30–60 minutes of aerobic exercise.

Thursday: 20–30 minutes of brisk walking plus the fat-burning and detox yoga programme.

Friday: 30–60 minutes of aerobic exercise.

Saturday: 30–45 minutes of walking plus the fat-burning and detox yoga programme.

Sunday: have a rest.

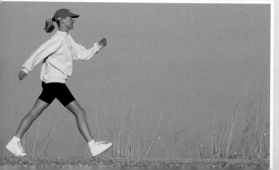

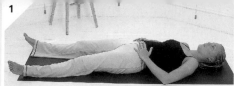

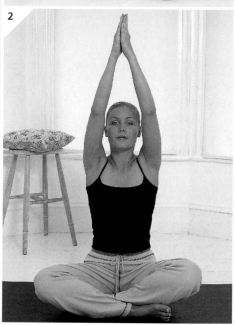

Fat-burning and detox yoga programme

This programme helps tone your muscles. You can do this with traditional exercise, but by using yoga moves you will also help calm the body and deal with the potentially stress-induced elements of weight gain.

1 **Yoga breathing.** Lie down with your legs straight, and press your lower back into the floor. If you find this hard, bend your knees. Put your fingers on your navel, and breathe in and out a few times. Next time when you inhale fill your lungs from the bottom upwards: so your tummy balloons out first and the chest last. Breathe in for a count of 5. Now exhale for a count of 10, letting the air out of the belly first, and the chest last. Repeat 5 times.

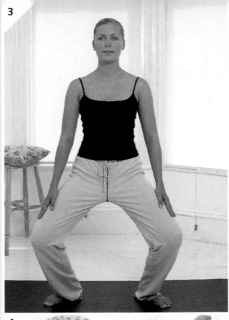

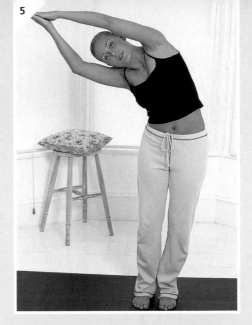

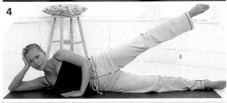

2 **Mountain pose**. Sit cross-legged and breathe in and out deeply. Inhale and stretch your arms up close to your ears and press your palms together. As you do this, your stomach muscles will pull in; hold the position for as long as you can and breathe regularly. Then exhale and bring your arms back to the starting position.

3 **Stick posture.** Stand with your feet about 25cm (10in) apart. Bend your knees as if you are preparing to sit, but then turn them slightly outwards. With your hands on your thighs, keep your torso as erect as you can and breathe in and out. Now exhale, and then pull your abdominal muscles back towards your navel and up towards your ribs. Hold this position until you need to breathe in, then inhale and straighten your body. Repeat once more.

4 **Side leg raise.** Lie on your side, supporting your head with one hand, and with the palm of the other hand on the floor to aid stability. Inhale and slowly raise your upper leg; it should come straight up, not slightly back or to the side. Also try not to bend the leg at the knee. Hold the leg in this position for as long as you possibly can, remembering not to hold your breath but breathing regularly. Exhale and lower your leg. Repeat this leg raise on the other side.

5 **Half-moon.** Stand up straight, with your feet together, and your arms by your sides. Inhale and bring your arms upwards, close to your ears, and press your palms together if you possibly can. Exhale and slowly bend to one side as far over as you can. Hold this position for as long as possible, breathing regularly as you do so. Return to the centre and repeat the process again, this time bending to the other side.

6 **Finish off.** Complete the programme by repeating the yoga breathing techniques from step 1.

FLUID-BUSTING MASSAGE

This massage should be carried out once a day. It aims to help the body eliminate fluid more effectively, stopping it from being reabsorbed into the tissues. It uses a very basic form of manual lymph drainage to do this, which means that instead of deep probing strokes you should use long, very gentle moves.

For best results, carry out the massage with a blend of essential oils that are designed to fight fat and fluid retention. For example, take two drops of grapefruit oil, two drops of mandarin oil and one drop of black pepper oil and add them to 10ml of carrier oil (test this first, since black pepper can irritate sensitive skins). You can also boost fluid loss by trying steams or saunas. Aim for one a week.

Start on your legs, at the ankles, moving upwards and towards the knees. Work both the front and the back of the body. Then move up the thighs, focusing upwards and towards the groin.

Work around the arms, moving upwards from wrist to elbow. Now move past the elbow, massaging the upper arms towards the armpit.

Now massage your torso. The area above your chest, the upper abdomen, should be massaged outwards and either up or down towards the armpits, depending on the area being treated. If someone is massaging your back, strokes on the upper back and shoulder blades should be towards the armpit; neck strokes towards the ears.

Work the lower abdomen. Anywhere under the area of your navel should be massaged down towards the groin. If someone is massaging your back, their strokes should go upwards.

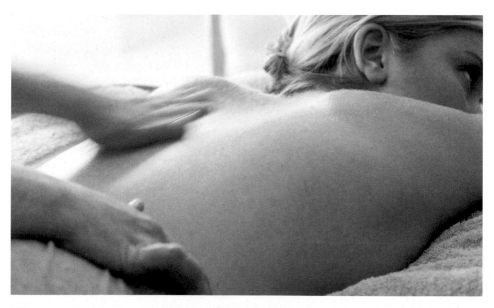

EXTENDING THE PLAN

If you get to the end of the month of the plan and still have more weight to lose, there's a good chance that it's fat that you now need to reduce, not fluid. You can therefore reintroduce wheat and dairy products into your diet in small amounts. Switch from soya to skimmed milk in breakfast meals. Add cottage cheese or 50g (2oz) of reduced-fat hard cheeses to your protein choices (and choose these once or twice a week). Also add wholegrain breads and wholewheat pastas to your carbohydrates in the evening (and again choose these once or twice a week). The rest of the diet stays the same.

You will also need to change the programme, because after a few weeks of carrying out the same activity the body begins to get used to exercises and they become less effective. The simplest way to beat this is to add intervals to the aerobic part of your plan. After every 2 minutes of normal aerobic activity, add 30 seconds to 2 minutes of working out at least 10 per cent faster. These mini energy bursts stimulate your body and stop it from getting 'bored'.

Living the detox life

If you've got to the end of the month and have lost all the weight you wanted to lose, that's great; but you need to make sure you don't put it back on again. Around 90 per cent of people who lose weight do just that, so here are some tips:

- Know your calorie count. If you eat more calories than you burn, you will gain weight no matter how cleansed your system is. To work out how many calories you can consume in a day without gaining weight, do this simple calculation.

Multiply your weight in kilograms by 0.9, then multiply this figure by 24. Multiply this third figure by one of the following: 1.3 if you are in a sedentary job and do no exercise; 1.5 if you are in a sedentary job but exercise for 1–3 hours a week; 1.7 if you are in a manual job or exercise heavily (for more than three hours a week). (For example, if you weigh 65kg and fall into the second category above, the calculation for your calorie intake would be: 65 x 0.9 = 58.5 x 24 = 1,404 x 1.5 = 2,106 kcals.)

- Start re-introducing wheat and dairy products. If you don't have a food intolerance, there is no point cutting out wheat and dairy products any longer. If you aren't sure, go back to normal levels but listen to your body: if you notice your waistline getting puffy or the scales adding 2kg (4lb) or more in a day, you have an intolerance. If this is the case, stay off them again for a few days, then introduce one to two servings of dairy foods and one to two servings of wheat foods daily. If you do keep dairy foods low, boost your calcium intake through leafy green vegetables such as spinach, kale and broccoli, calcium-enriched products like orange juice and bony fish like sardines. (The body needs calcium to burn fat.)

- Reduce your toxic load. If you didn't follow the advice for the Anti-pollution Plan (see page 52), go back and do just that. It'll also help to drink the Chelating Cocktail (see page 53) daily from now on.

- Keep exercising. According to the US National Weight Registry (the world's biggest survey of people who have successfully lost weight) exercise is the key. The average person, in their studies, burns 2,800 calories a week through exercise – that's a daily walk of 5–6km (3–4 miles). Make this your aim too.

beauty-boosting plan

Most of us have days when we look in the mirror and simply despair of our appearance. This is the plan for those depressing moments. It'll instantly re-energize your skin and your hair, making them look much healthier, and also offers tips to help strengthen both of these in the future.

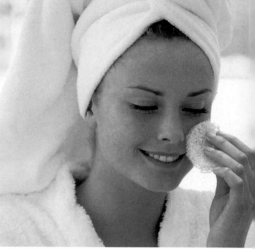

About skin and toxins

Skin is one of the first parts of the body to show problems from toxic overload.

The main reason for this is that the body sees it as a non-essential organ; therefore, if toxins are wreaking havoc on the rest of the body, destroying nutrient stores and such like, the body diverts nutrients away from the skin to allow it to supply them to more vital organs like the heart and lungs. This is bad news for our looks, because the skin relies completely on nutrients for its health; if it's lacking in essential fatty acids that the body has diverted to the brain, for example, it will appear dry and lack lustre.

SMOKING

Toxins can attack our skin in other ways, too. The healthy look of the skin depends on the circulation being able to supply it with the nutrients and oxygen it needs. Many toxins interfere with this process –

the worst one being smoking, which constricts blood vessels and causes smokers to have a sallow, yellow complexion. On top of this, it's been shown in research that smokers in their 40s have the same number of wrinkles as non-smokers 20 years older. This happens, according to doctors at Nagoya City University Medical School in Japan, because smoking increases levels in the body of an enzyme called matrix metalloproteinase (MMP), the job of which is to break down collagen – the fibre that keeps the skin firm.

ALCOHOL

Another toxin that causes problems with the skin is alcohol; in the body this is broken down into acetaldehyde. This chemical first attacks collagen and elastin, but also alters the shape of the red blood cells circulating in the blood, thereby reducing the amount of oxygen travelling around the system.

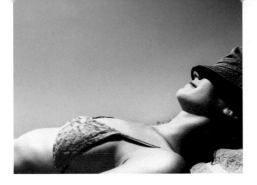

hair growth by 10 per cent through massaging and stimulating the scalp; it's not difficult to see, then, that poor circulation could impede growth by at least this much. Finally, hair has its own toxins to handle, such as perming lotions, chemical dyes, harsh shampoos and heat from blow-dryers. All of these are 'toxic' to the hair.

STRESS

Stress can trigger dull-looking skin because it wipes out the B vitamins our circulation needs to create healthy red blood cells.

SUNLIGHT

When it comes to our skin, the real toxin is the sun. Dermatologists estimate that if we didn't expose our skin to the sun we wouldn't get a wrinkle until we were 60. As it is, most of us start to see the first sign of ageing in our early 30s, if not before.

Sunlight causes problems because it allows high levels of free radicals to be formed in the skin, and these start to attack the collagen and elastin fibres that keep our skin firm. Just 4 minutes of sun exposure is enough to start this whole process happening. Sunlight also thickens the upper layers of the skin, which creates an unfortunate, dull, sallow appearance.

About hair and toxins

Toxins can also cause hair to look dry and dull, for the same reasons as skin – it's not seen as an essential organ.

If the body decides the muscles need more B vitamins (because they are under stress), these will be diverted away from hair, cutting the supply of the fuel it needs to grow. Hair growth is also affected by poor circulation. It's been shown that you boost

The solution

Detoxing your skin and hair is therefore a matter of reducing many of these toxins, or at the very least strengthening them against them (how to do the latter is explained in the second part of the plan).

However, in the short term, you can dramatically improve the look of your skin and hair with intensive treatments, plus massage and other moves that boost circulation. So the plan starts with an instant-result programme to stop 'bad mirror days' in their tracks.

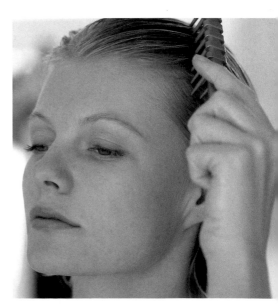

Instant-result programme

Carry out the following regime once to improve the look of your skin and hair instantly; then use the elements marked with an asterisk (*) nightly to fight beauty problems for good.

1 **Shampoo your hair.** Then towel dry it so it is just damp. Apply an intensive conditioning treatment or mix up your own with half a cup of warm (not hot) olive oil and ten drops of lavender essential oil. Apply this to the hair using gentle massage movements to stimulate the scalp. Once the hair is coated, tie a plastic carrier bag around your hair (obviously keeping your face well clear) to increase the rate at which the treatment penetrates the hair. Leave this on while you carry out your facial.

2 ***The 'Lion'.** It may sound bizarre to start a facial with some yoga, but this move actually tones your facial muscles while reducing muscle tension that can hinder circulation. Sit comfortably on the floor or a chair, resting your palms on your legs. Inhale, then exhale slowly; while you do this, open your eyes and mouth as wide as possible. Very slowly, stick your tongue out and down as far as it will go (without straining), and you'll feel the muscles around your face tighten. Now stiffen your arms and fingers. Hold this position for as long as you can, then slowly relax.

3 ***Cleansing Cleanse.** Use your normal cleanser, or mix up a natural cleanser using a tablespoonful of natural yogurt and a teaspoonful of lemon juice. Dab this off the skin with a tissue, then rinse with cool water.

4 **Exfoliate the skin.** Use a gentle store-bought exfoliator to do this, or, alternatively, add enough water to a teaspoon of sugar to make it into a smooth paste – make sure that it isn't too thick and scratchy or too liquid.

5 **Steam the skin.** Steaming helps release any toxins and impurities that may be just under the skin's surface, blocking circulation. Fill a bowl with boiling water, then gently place your face about 10cm (4in) from the surface and hold for 2–3 minutes. You can intensity the effects of the steam by placing a towel over your head to trap the vapours, but don't do this if you have asthma because it can irritate the respiratory tract.

6 ***Splash the skin.** Using cold water, quickly splash the skin 20–30 times with water. Then pat it dry with a towel. On a night when you haven't steamed the skin, you can even do this with iced water to rapidly boost the blood flow to the area; ice

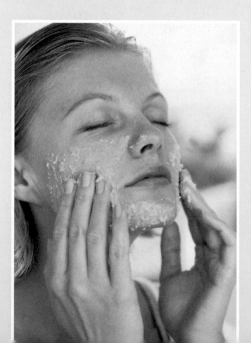

is best avoided on steam nights, though, as the dramatic change in temperature can over-stress the skin, leading to broken veins.

(7) ***Add moisture.** Now it's time to moisturize the face. On ordinary nights, you can do this with your normal moisturizer, using the same moves; but on this programme you're going to use essential oils because these can create rapid improvements to the skin's surface. Apply two drops of your chosen oil (use camomile for dry skins, rose for oily skins, and carrotseed for mature skins) to a carrier oil. Grapeseed is a great oil to use, since it's fine enough to use on the face and has antioxidant properties; if you're pregnant, just use the grapeseed oil. Now apply the moisturizer, massaging the skin as you go.

- Start at your chin, gently smoothing the skin upwards with the pads of your fingers; don't tug the skin, just smooth it gently. Now drum your fingers lightly again, moving upwards up the jaw line. Repeat 5 times.

- Repeat these moves over your cheeks. Now quickly pat the cheeks and jaw 5–10 times; start lightly but then get firmer.
- Stroke up around the temples and up the forehead. Repeat the drumming motion.
- When you get to the middle of the forehead, use alternate index fingers to brush rapidly upwards from the middle of your brows to the hairline; this should feel like a smooth rolling movement.
- Finally, treat the under-eye area. Dab a little oil along the socket bone below your eye (oils should never go directly on the eye area), and massage this in well, using gentle upward strokes. Finish by lightly drumming your fingers along the socket bone. Repeat the process under your other eye.

(8) **Rinse off your hair.** This may take a couple of shampoos and then apply conditioner. Rinse again and towel dry. If you have to blow-dry, use warm air, not hot, and keep the dryer as far away from the hair as possible.

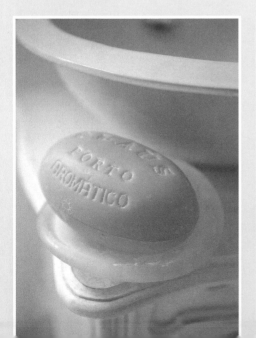
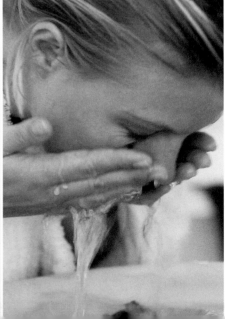

Your hair and skin's needs

needs

doesn't need

SKIN

Antioxidants. These are the most vital way to protect your skin against free-radical attack. Studies at the University of Arizona, USA, have found that eating at least six servings of red or yellow vegetables a day is actually the same as wearing sun-protection factor (SPF) 4 on your skin in its ability to protect you against sun damage. Aim for six to ten servings of fresh fruit or vegetables a day for best results. This will also supply vitamin C, which helps build collagen, and vitamin A, which encourages the growth of new skin cells.

Essential fatty acids. As well as keeping red blood cells healthy, which boosts circulation, essential fatty acids also help fight dry skin. Good sources are oily fish, nuts and seeds – aim for one serving a day.

Sulphur. This helps the body form new collagen. You'll find it in eggs, onions and garlic. Aim for one serving a day.

Sugar. As well as being a major source of free radicals, sugar also attacks the skin. It attaches to proteins in collagen and this causes them to become stiff and inflexible, eventually leading to wrinkling.

Salty foods. These are high in iodine, which can encourage the skin to break out.

HAIR

B vitamins. Hair doesn't grow unless adequate levels of B vitamins are found in the body. You'll find them in wholegrains, dairy products, leafy green vegetables. Aim for at least three servings a day.

Essential fatty acids. Like skin, a lack of these fatty acids creates dry hair. Have at least one serving (see above) daily.

Protein. If we don't get enough protein in our diet, hair actually grows with a lifted cuticle. This not only increases the risk of dehydration, but it also makes hair look dull because light can't reflect from it. Aim for two servings of protein-rich foods (like eggs, fish, dairy products, nuts, pulses or meat) each day.

Vitamin H (biotin). Found in eggs, fish, milk, nuts and pulses, this nutrient actually helps hair (and nails) grow. Aim for one serving of biotin-rich foods a day.

Too much vitamin A. While this nutrient may help skin, high quantities of foods that are heavy in vitamin A, like liver, can actually trigger hair loss; instead, get your vitamin A through foods containing beta-carotene (like carrots, pumpkin, sweet potatoes), since this doesn't cause the same reaction.

EATING YOUR WAY TO GOOD HAIR AND SKIN

Like so many elements of our health, what we eat can make the difference between good skin and hair and dull, dry versions. Skin and hair need slightly different things to thrive (see chart opposite), but this diet will aid both.

A DAY'S DIET AT A GLANCE

- Start by taking a multivitamin and mineral supplement, plus 1,000mg of methyl sulfonyl methane (which converts to sulphur in the body) and 500mg of evening primrose oil. Drink at least one glass of water, and aim to drink another eight throughout the day.
- For breakfast, have a bowl of bran or wheat cereal topped with skimmed milk, two tablespoons of blueberries and two of raspberries. Drink a glass of orange juice.
- Mid-morning, have a piece of fruit and a handful of nuts or a low-fat yogurt.
- At lunchtime, take another 500mg of evening primrose oil. Have a sandwich of two slices of wholegrain bread filled with 50g (2oz) fish, chicken or low-fat cheese. Top with lettuce or alfalfa sprouts, chopped onion, tomato, avocado and cucumber. Serve with a cup of tomato, carrot or vegetable soup.
- Mid-afternoon, eat a piece of fruit.
- Before your evening meal, take another 500mg of evening primrose oil.
- For your meal, eat a 75g (3oz) serving of lean protein. Serve with 50g (2oz) brown rice, wholewheat pasta, jacket potato, new potatoes or wholegrain bread. Add equal amounts of a green vegetable and another vegetable.

Living the detox life

As well as integrating the diet advice into your normal life, there are three other essentials for good looks:

- Use sunscreen. This is the most vital thing that you can ever do for your skin. You should apply at least an SPF 15 sunscreen 30 minutes before you go into the sun; even in winter, ultraviolet rays still break through clouds. If you have sensitive skin, screens that use titanium dioxide as a block may cause fewer problems than so-called chemical sunscreens. Hair should also be protected with sun-protective sprays because sunlight dries it out.
- Stop smoking with the Stop Smoking Plan given on page 82.
- Keep your skincare regime simple. If a product has more than ten ingredients, it could make your skin sensitive. Stick to products with short ingredient lists and keep the amount you use to a minimum. Even the most mature skin needs only a cleanser, a moisturizer, a vitamin C serum for the daytime and a vitamin A cream at night – plus sunscreen, of course.

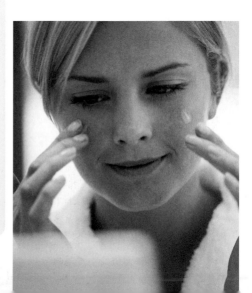

anti-cellulite plan

If anyone needs to describe cellulite to you, then you probably don't need this plan! If, however, you're personally familiar with this lumpy, bumpy, bulging type of skin, then read on. It is possible to detox your cellulite through a combination of diet, exercise and certain external treatments.

About cellulite and toxins

In the past few years, a common theory on cellulite has been that it is caused by toxins collecting under the skin.

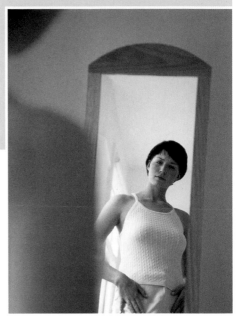

This is not true. No one has even found debris of caffeine in cellulite when they've measured it; nor have they found nicotine, alcohol or the remnants of the cheeseburger eaten ten years ago. While toxins may play a role in the formation of cellulite, they are not the problem. The truth is that cellulite is just fat, much the same as what's on your the rest of your body. What's different about cellulite, and the reason why it has that lumpy, bumpy, orange-peel appearance, however, is how that fat is held in place.

All around the exterior of the body, there is a layer of fat under the skin called the subcutis. It keeps us warm, it cushions us when we sit down and it protects our bones. Through this layer run fibres of collagen that collect the fat into pockets. Normally, these fibres are thin and the pockets remain smooth; however, changes can occur to this. The fat becomes damaged and lumpy, and instead of being thin and smooth the collagen fibres start to thicken, pressing into the fat and creating bulging. It is this unsightly bulging, which we all hate, that is cellulite.

WHY DOES THIS HAPPEN?

As yet, no one really knows why, but it's increasingly looking as if two factors play a big role. The first is free-radical attack. Free radicals attack the healthy cells of the body, and this is also true of fat cells. As well as this, free radicals have a particular affinity for collagen and elastin fibres that make up the top layers of the skin. When these tissues degrade, the skin thins and this reduces the covering over the subcutis, making the (now bumpy) fat layer underneath more noticeable.

The second factor is sluggish blood circulation and lymph flow. The job of the circulation is to carry nutrients to the cells of the body, while the lymph carries away toxic byproducts. If these things aren't working correctly, they can compound the problem. According to leading cellulite researcher Elisabeth Dancey, author of *The Cellulite Solution* (Hodder and Stoughton, 1996), when skin cells called fibroblasts are deprived of oxygen they start to clump together. So, during repair of the damaged collagen, these cells create thick, stringy fibres instead of thin, healthy ones. Furthermore, she says that if lymph flow is slow, the fluid solidifies and creates thick fibres of its own. These two processes then create thick strands that make fat bulge.

The solution

Beating cellulite is a three-step process. First you need to reduce fat in the cellulite area (and disguise what doesn't get reduced); second, reduce and repair free-radical damage and finally boost blood circulation and lymph flow.

By combining diet, exercise and external treatments for six to eight weeks, you can dramatically reduce the look of any cellulite.

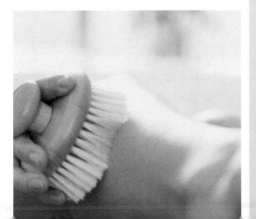

Anti-cellulite diet

Cellulite can be difficult to shift, but if you follow the following rules, you will maximize your body's chances of reducing those tell-tale dimples.

FIVE MAIN RULES APPLY

1 **Eat your antioxidants.** These are our number one defence against free radicals and are found in all fruits and vegetables. On the diet you should be aiming for at least five servings of fruit and vegetables a day. A serving constitutes: two tablespoons of vegetables; a 250g (8oz) slice of large fruits like watermelon; two tablespoons of small fruits like berries; and one piece of medium fruit like apples. As well as this, the antioxidant vitamins C and E play a part in strengthening the skin, and so you should take supplements of these. Take 3g of vitamin C (the most your body can store) in three 1g doses, daily, and 400iu of vitamin E daily.

2 **Use other skin strengtheners.** Foods other than fruit and vegetables have also been shown to have antioxidant properties – wholemeal cereals, for example. Green tea is also a powerful source and is essential in an anti-cellulite diet. Studies at the University of Geneva, Switzerland, have found that it boosts metabolism, while French researchers have revealed that green tea cuts by a third the release of enzymes that cause the body to store fat. Drink at least three cups daily. Finally, according to research at the University of Pavia, Italy the herb gotu kola triggers the formation of healthy collagen, but does this without increasing numbers of water-attracting cells (which is good news). Take 30mg three times daily.

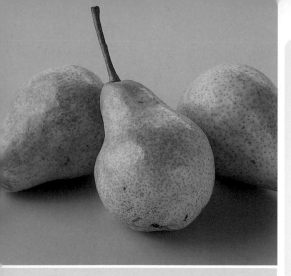

3 **Supplement your circulation.** The herb ginkgo biloba is used in many anti-cellulite creams, but taking it internally also boosts circulation. The recommended dose is 120mg a day. Foods containing essential fatty acids also help aid circulation, so oily fish, nuts, seeds and oils such as flaxseed should be a daily part of the plan.

4 **Eat some low-fat protein at every mealtime.** Cellulite contains higher than normal quantities of water-attracting cells, which is bad news when circulation and lymph flow are blocked since this causes fluid to leak from cells and get trapped in surrounding tissues. Protein, however, contains a substance called albumin that helps prevent this leakage, helping reduce the fluid levels. Drinking plenty of water and cutting out salty foods will also help here.

5 **Reduce your fat and sugar content.** Both of these add to the free-radical load your skin is under, but high-fat and high-sugar foods are also loaded with calories. The more calories you eat the higher your chance of weight gain – and, remember, cellulite is just plain fat.

ONE DAY'S DIET AT A GLANCE

- Early on take 1g of vitamin C, 400iu of vitamin E, 120mg of ginkgo biloba and 30mg of gotu kola with a glass of water. Drink water every hour.
- For breakfast, eat a bowl of bran cereal with skimmed milk. Top with a chopped banana and strawberries. Drink a glass of orange juice.
- Mid-morning, have a cup of green tea and two pieces of fluid-filled fruit (watermelon, pears or grapes).
- At lunchtime, take 1g of vitamin C and 30mg of gotu kola. Eat a salad of leafy green vegetables (rocket, baby spinach, alfalfa sprouts, shredded green cabbage, broccoli), topped with red vegetables (tomatoes, red onions, beetroot, red peppers), yellow/orange vegetables (carrots, yellow peppers) and white vegetables (radish, white cabbage, onions). This gives the ultimate mix of antioxidants. Add 75g (3oz) of lean protein: chicken, fish (especially oily fish like tuna, mackerel, salmon), lean ham, beans, tofu, sunflower seeds or nuts. Also include a teaspoon of flaxseed oil.
- Mid-afternoon, have two more pieces of fruit with a low-fat yogurt. Drink another cup of green tea.
- At dinner time, take 1g of vitamin C and 30mg of gotu kola. Have 75g (3oz) of lean protein with 75g (3oz) of carbohydrates: wholewheat pasta, brown rice, jacket or new potatoes, couscous or wholegrain, rye or pumpernickel breads. Serve with two portions of any vegetables.
- Before bed, try to drink another cup of green tea.

Anti-cellulite exercise programme

Exercise is vital in beating cellulite. It burns calories to reduce fat, boosts circulation and lymph drainage, and can also help disguise cellulite by increasing muscle tone under the skin. The following regime should be carried out for the six weeks of the plan.

Monday: 30–60 minutes of aerobic exercise such as walking, running, rowing, cycling or dancing.
Tuesday: tone and detox programme (see below).
Wednesday: 30–60 minutes of aerobic exercise.
Thursday: tone and detox programme.
Friday: 30–60 minutes of aerobic exercise.
Saturday: tone and detox programme.
Sunday: have a rest.

TONE AND DETOX PROGRAMME

The following programme combines strength training moves to boost tone in the hips and thighs, but also uses yoga moves to help stimulate lymph flow and blood circulation. Some of the moves say to use dumbbells or weights: this isn't essential, but it will improve your results.

1 **Warm up.** Spend 10 minutes walking, jogging, skipping, dancing or, if you have a mini-trampoline, rebounding, to warm up your body.

2 **Squats.** You will need a dumbbell (or other suitable weight, such as a tin of baked beans or similar) – about 4–7kg (9–15lb) is best. Standing up straight, with your feet hip-width apart, hold the dumbbell (or other weight) between your legs, with your arms straight. Keeping your arms as they are (they move with you), squat down as if you were going to sit in a chair. Make sure that you do this with your bottom muscles, not by widening your legs; your knees mustn't go further forward than your ankle. Now use your thigh/buttock muscles to push yourself back up to a standing position. When you reach the top, clench your bottom and hold for 1 second. Do this 12 times; then repeat the whole sequence 4 times.

3 **Wide squats.** Stand up straight with your feet more than hip-width apart; they should be wider than in Squats. Turn your feet out to so that they're at a 45-degree angle. Perform the same squatting movement as before, watching your knees again. Do 4 sets of 12 repetitions.

2
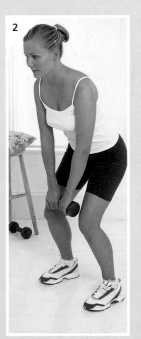

3
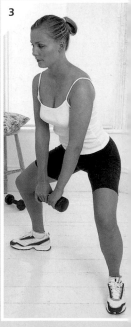

117

4

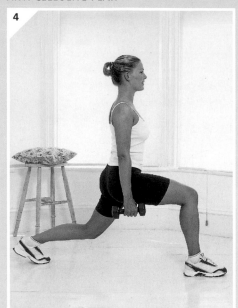

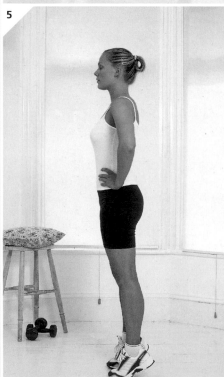

4 **Lunges.** Hold a dumbbell (or other weight) in each hand, resting your arms by your side. Now take a step forward and, as you do this, dip down so the other knee bends towards the floor, and your body goes with it. Focus on ensuring your knee does not go further forward than your ankle and that your feet don't turn, which reduces the effect. Push up from the foot on your bent leg (you should feel it in your bottom and inner thigh) and come back to the standing position. Do 12 movements, then repeat on the other leg. Do the whole sequence 4 times.

5 **Calf raises.** Stand up straight with your feet flat on the floor, but turned so your toes are pointing slightly towards each other. Raise up onto your toes, tensing your calf muscles. Slowly lower back down. Do 4 sets of 12 repetitions.

6 **Leg vibrations.** Lie on your back and put your legs in the air. Open them so they are hip-width apart, then tense your legs and try to find a point at which they naturally start to vibrate. Let yourself 'wobble' for up to 2 minutes.

5

6

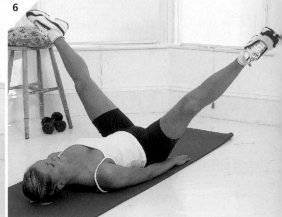

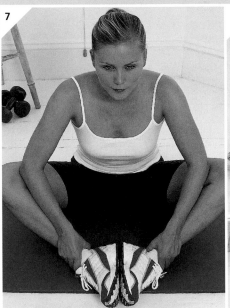

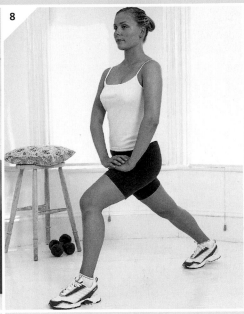

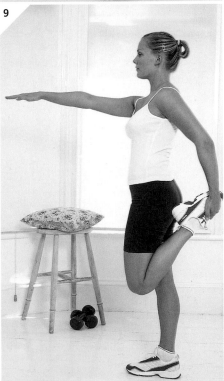

7 **Butterfly.** Sit on the floor with your legs apart, knees bent and the soles of your feet together. Rest your hands on your ankles, arms by your sides. Exhale and, as you do this, bring your knees upwards so they press against your arms. Inhale and press them back down. Do this 10 times.

8 **Calf stretch.** Step forward with your left leg and bend your knee. As you do this, your right leg will straighten and your heel will come off the floor. Keeping this leg straight, try to push your heel back down gently. Hold for 30 seconds when you feel the stretch. Release and swap legs.

9 **Thigh stretch.** Stand up straight. Lift your left ankle up behind you. Grasp your foot and gently try to pull it to touch your bottom. Hold this stretch in your thigh for 30 seconds, putting out your arm for balance if you need to. Lower, then repeat on the other leg.

EXTERNAL TREATMENTS

Every day you should carry out body-brushing (see page 28) as part of the anti-cellulite programme. Once you've finished body-brushing, and after any bath or shower you take, you should apply an external cellulite treatment. No matter what the hype tells you, these will not melt away your cellulite. Instead, you're aiming to plump up the dermis using moisturizing ingredients (which helps disguise the cellulite), to firm and tone the skin and to boost circulation. Look for creams that contain one or more of the following ingredients:

Retinol. This is possibly the most important, since it has been clinically proven to improve skin tone.

Horse chestnut. This has been used in research trials to strengthen weakened veins and boost circulation.

Gotu kola. This helps build healthy collagen when taken as a supplement and may also work externally.

Caffeine. This works as a diuretic, but may also trigger enzymes that switch on cells that cause fat to be released.

Aminophylline. This may also help promote fat-burning; it's certainly been shown to shrink thighs.

If you would prefer to use aromatherapy oils to treat your cellulite, choose oils that strengthen the skin and decrease fluid. A good blend would be: one drop of fennel (do not use this if you are epileptic), one drop of cypress, one drop of grapefruit and two drops of juniper, added to 10ml of carrier oil. Use this for a massage or put it in a warm bath. (Do not use this blend of oils if you're pregnant.)

Apply your chosen treatment to the affected areas in an upward motion. Don't knead and press the skin in an attempt to squeeze down the cellulite. This can damage the skin further and also doesn't aid the lymph flow or the circulation. When rubbing anything into your legs, always use long, gentle strokes. Also carry out a weekly lymph massage (see page 106).

Use sunscreen. Having a tan disguises cellulite, but sunlight is the number one degrader of collagen and elastin fibres. Just 4 minutes of sun exposure in high summer can be shown to break them down. If you must have a tan, use a fake one.

Living the detox life

If you follow this programme for six weeks, you should notice a distinct difference in the amount and severity of your cellulite. You can then continue the programme further to see more benefits, or, if you're happy, follow the advice given here – sadly, getting rid of your cellulite doesn't mean it won't come back if you don't keep things up.

- Continue to eat at least five portions of fruit and vegetables a day, and take 1g of vitamin C and 400iu of vitamin E daily.
- Get at least 30 minutes of activity daily. This could be formal exercise, or it could just be running up and down the stairs instead of taking the lift.
- Monitor your weight. Don't be obsessive, but if you gain more than 1–1.5kg (2–3lb) cut back on high-calorie foods to stop things in their tracks. The easiest way to lose weight without realizing you're on a diet is to eat what you normally eat but serve yourself 25 per cent less of everything (except fruit and vegetables).
- Use at least an SPF15 sunscreen whenever you go into the sun.

live longer plan

There is no particular 'right' time to implement this plan. Instead, it's the one you should put into practice generally in your everyday life, whatever age you are now, if you want to give yourself the maximum chance of living a long, healthy and fulfilling life.

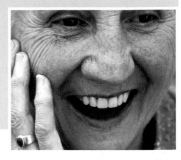

About lifespan and toxins

The number of people living to over 100 in the world is increasing. In 1955, the Queen sent 300 birthday telegrams to British subjects reaching their centenary; in the year 2000 she would have penned over 8,000. In the USA in 1900 only one in every 100,000 citizens reached 100, but today one in every 10,000 makes the milestone. In fact, it's estimated that, by the year 2030, there will be 30,000 centenarians in the UK alone, and, by 2050, 1 million in the USA.

The reason for this is partly that our improved medical knowledge is helping defeat diseases that would have ended lives sooner, and partly that our own personal knowledge about what is good for us means many of us are living healthier lives.

GENETIC FACTORS

How long we live is predominantly controlled by our ageing genes. It's believed that about ten major genes are responsible for ageing, and that what causes us to get old is changes in functions in these genes. For example, studies at the University of Wisconsin, USA, have found that as we get older genes that help create cell and DNA

damage double in activity, while those that control tissue regeneration reduce their activity by half. This means that, day by day, cells start to get destroyed and your body doesn't repair them as well, which eventually leads to deterioration of major systems like the brain, heart and lungs. You may be thinking 'If it's programmed into my system, how can I try to fight ageing?' Experts believe that the human body should be able to live to 100–120 years of age; and what stops this happening is the way we live our lives, with exposure to toxins playing a major role.

TOXINS AND AGEING

Toxins have the ability to switch on our ageing genes faster than nearly anything else. The reason for this is those free radicals once again. These are the number one cause of ageing, triggering everything from wrinkles to the atherosclerosis that causes heart disease, and mutations in the cells that can cause cancer. Epidemiological studies (where huge numbers of the population are studied for trends) have found that: vegetarians live an average of seven years longer than average; non-smokers (or people who have given up long-term) live five to seven years longer than smokers; men who take supplements of vitamin C live six years longer than those who don't; and people who stick to one to two alcoholic drinks a day live five years longer than those regularly drinking more than this, or who don't drink at all. What all these behaviours have in common is that they expose your body to lower levels of free radicals than eating meat, smoking or drinking large amounts of alcohol do.

So, put simply, by carrying out some small changes to your lifestyle now, you could potentially detox your life against ageing in the future. These changes don't even need to be particularly radical, as you'll see in this final (but most vital) plan.

The solution

The Live Longer Plan is divided into two parts: diet and lifestyle. Unlike the other plans, there is no one-day, six-week or even six-month plan to boost longevity. Instead here are live-longer tips that will help extend your life if made a part of your everyday life.

How you use this plan is up to you. You can radically change your life, incorporating all the elements in one go; or you can make it an ongoing project, aiming to incorporate one tip a month for the next year or two. Whatever you do, it will help.

'People who stick to one to two alcoholic drinks a day live five years longer than those regularly drinking more than this.'

Live longer diet rules

If you follow these rules, you will increase your chances of leading not only a longer life, but a healthier one with fewer age related diseases.

1 **REDUCE YOUR CALORIES**
A low-calorie, high-nutrient diet has been shown to prevent 84 per cent of the major gene changes that occur in ageing. 'High-nutrient' means based primarily on fruit and vegetables and wholegrain carbohydrates, with low (if any) levels of everything else. But what does 'low-calorie' mean?

According to research by the Arizona College of Medicine, USA, going as low as 900–1,100 calories a day could extend your lifespan by up to 15 years; but other studies have shown that just cutting calories by 25 per cent will aid the average person. That means consuming a total of around 1,500 calories a day for the average woman and around 2,000 for the average man.

2 **EAT LESS FAT**
No more than 30 per cent of your daily calories should come from fat, with less than 10 per cent of these coming from saturated fats. This is the key to a longer life – according to just about every heart health organization in the world. It's also been shown that low-fat diets reduce the risk of colon and rectal cancers and may lower the risk of breast, ovarian and prostate cancers.

The impact of beating cancer and heart disease has massive effects on longevity: according to the American Academy for Anti-Aging Medicine, doing so will add an average of 13 years to your overall lifespan.

To work out how much fat you can safely eat in a day, look at how many calories you eat in a day (see page 107), then calculate 30 per cent of this. Now divide this figure by 9 (which is the number of calories in 1g of fat). This tells you how many grams of fat you can eat a day without any harm to your health; saturated fat (like that found in animal fats) should make up less than a third of these.

3 EAT LESS SUGAR

Aim for less than 40g (1½oz) of sugar a day. Not only is it a major cause of free radicals, but it's also linked to increased risk of Type II diabetes, and this condition can knock 20 years off your lifespan.

4 EAT MORE THAN FIVE SERVINGS OF FRUIT AND VEGETABLES A DAY

These are our best defence against free radicals, and as such it's believed that at least five servings a day could increase life expectancy by 15 years. The top 10 antioxidant-filled fruits are: prunes, raisins, blueberries, blackberries, strawberries, raspberries, plums, oranges, red grapes and cherries. The top 10 antioxidant-filled vegetables are: kale, spinach, brussels sprouts, alfalfa sprouts, broccoli florets, beets, red peppers, onion, corn and aubergine.

5 GO VEGETARIAN

Vegetarians live up to seven years longer than meat-eaters, according to research from Linda University, California, USA. As yet, no one knows why. It could be because vegetarian diets include more fibre; but it could be because of a high intake of fruits and vegetables or lowered levels of animal fats. If you can give up eating meat – or at least dramatically cut down – you will certainly improve your health.

6 DRINK TEA

It's an additional way of getting antioxidants into the body and has been shown to aid heart health by researchers at Harvard University, USA. Two cups a day extended life by at least three years. Green tea, oolong tea and black tea were all shown to provide benefits.

7 EAT GARLIC

Taking garlic supplements every day from your 30s onwards makes your heart behave as if it were 13 years younger, says research from the Centre for Cardiovascular Pharmacology in Mainz, Germany. The reason for this is that, as the heart ages, the arteries around it stiffen. This slows the speed at which the blood pumps around

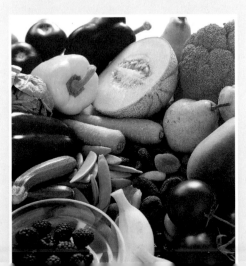
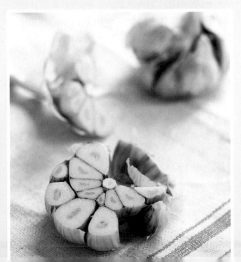

the body, increasing the risk of heart attack. Garlic seems to stop this happening, potentially due to its high antioxidant count. So you should eat fresh garlic at least once a day, but also supplement this with a garlic tablet or capsule.

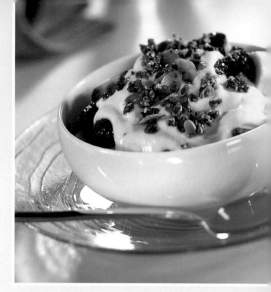

8 BOOST YOUR DETOX ENZYMES

Adding at least four to five of the top detox foods (see pages 17–19) will maximize your body's ability to neutralize harmful toxins that may cause damage in the body. Researchers at the University of Michigan, USA have already found that people who live the longest also have the highest levels of the detox substance glutathione in their body; boosting all the detox processes could therefore add even greater benefits.

9 MAKE SURE YOU EAT BREAKFAST

Breakfast cereals contain high levels of folic acid, which research from Leeds University, UK has shown lowers the levels of an amino acid called homocysteine in the body. Doctors believe that this artery-clogging substance may actually be more harmful to us than cholesterol.

10 EAT CHOCOLATE

Yes, you read that right. Studies by the Harvard School of Public Health, USA, have shown that chocolate-eaters live longer than those who give up sweets completely. The reason is that chocolate contains exceptionally high levels of antioxidants. Many of us also use chocolate to calm us down and fighting stress is another way to live longer. Aim for two small squares daily, and opt for chocolate that is high (over 70 per cent) in cocoa solids.

At-a-glance diet guide

All this means that your daily diet should contain the following.

• At least five servings of fruit and vegetables, but ideally go for ten, four or five of which should be good detox foods (see pages 17–19).
• Three to four 75g (3oz) servings of wholegrain carbohydrates, one of which should be a high-fibre breakfast cereal fortified with folic acid.
• No more than one serving of meat, poultry or fish.
• No more than one serving of low-fat dairy produce (such as milk or cheese). Switch to calcium-enriched soya milk instead.
• One or two alcoholic drinks, preferably red wine.
• One garlic supplement and a multivitamin.
• Two squares of chocolate.

Live longer lifestyle

Living longer is not just about what you eat. There are a number of plans in this book that can help. As well as all the advice in these, there are a few other things to take into account.

EXERCISE

Exercise prolongs life. It lowers blood pressure, strengthens the heart, decreases body fat and lowers stress levels. It's been estimated that 4–5 hours of vigorous exercise, such as running, a week, adds three years to your life; but, if you're not a lover of the gym, burning 1,500 calories a week through gentle exercise like gardening or walking also adds at least a year.

THINK POSITIVE

Optimists normally live ten years longer than pessimists. This is because negative emotions depress our immune systems, making us more prone to illness. The immune system plays a vital role in fighting ageing: it fights changes in cells that can potentially turn cancerous. The problem is that the immune system has a finite life, and the more minor bugs it's exposed to the less it can fight against serious problems in later life. Keeping your immune system healthy is another way to extend your life – check the Good Health Plan (see page 96).

KEEP YOUR BRAIN ACTIVE

One thing that people who reach the age of 100 have in common is an active mind. The brain can develop new brain cells at any age and this has been linked to a reduced risk of problems like Alzheimer's disease. Keeping your brain active will help keep it healthy, but to build new neurones you also need to challenge the brain. One of the best ways to do this involves exercises called neurobics, where you carry out simple tasks in a different way – brushing your teeth with the 'wrong' hand, or driving home a different way each night.

FIND SOCIAL SUPPORT

Social support is another thing that centenarians have in common. On average, having six good friends who you can call on seems to have the best results. Stress relief seems to be the main benefit on the body: if you have someone to talk to when times get tough, you're less likely to succumb to toxic harm. If you find it hard to make friends, get a pet.

USE MEDICAL TECHNOLOGY

Health checks, like mammograms or cervical smears for women, or prostate or testicular checks for men, catch health problems much earlier, and the earlier cancers are found the greater the success rates of treatments. It is also important to have heart health checks: if you have high blood pressure and/or cholesterol, you can tackle these problems so they cause less damage.

Living the detox life

Every tip in this plan helps you live the detox life when it comes to longevity. It truly is a plan for life, but remember – life is meant to be enjoyed. Don't spend so long trying to improve your health that you don't enjoy every day you have – even the longest life is too short to be wasted.

index

acid balance, 37, 84
acupressure, 46, 59, 71, 79, 101
addiction, 57, 82–4
adrenaline, 66, 70
aerobic exercise, 20–1, 94
ageing, 109, 121–5
agnus castus, 99
air pollution, 48–9, 50–2
alcohol, 6, 7, 8, 12, 14
    and ageing, 122
    effects on skin, 108
    and immune system, 96
    Post-party Hangover Plan, 78–81
    Pre-party Plan, 74–7
    Sugar-busting Plan, 63
    and weight gain, 100
alfalfa, 19
alkaline foods, 84
allergies, 40, 67, 96, 98
amino acids, 75, 80, 124
aminophylline, 120
ammonia, 94
angelica oil, 36
antioxidant cocktail, 101, 102
antioxidants, 11, 17, 18, 19, 21, 52–3, 74, 100, 112, 115
appetite, 87, 93, 101
apples, 17
aromatherapy see essential oils
arteries, 123–4
arthritis, 67, 74
artichokes, 17
artificial sweeteners, 63
asparagus, 19
aubergine and tofu bake, 53
auto-immune diseases, 67, 96
avocados, 17, 54

Bach flower remedies, 71, 88
back massage, 32–3
bacteria, in bowel, 10, 40
bananas, 19
baths, 35, 45, 47, 95
Beauty-boosting Plan, 108–13
beauty products, 51
beetroot, 17–18
bentonite baths, 55
beta-carotene, 19, 97
biotin, 112
black pepper oil, 34, 36, 88
blood circulation, 23, 29, 30, 66, 74, 82, 91, 109, 115, 123–4
blood pressure, 21, 68, 125

blood-sugar levels, 14, 46, 58, 62, 63, 78, 80, 88, 90–1, 93
body-brushing, 28–9, 92, 120
body temperature, 13, 30, 98
bowel, 11
    bacteria, 10, 40
    constipation, 13, 40, 41, 87
    transit times, 20, 40
brain, ageing, 125
bran cereals, 19
Brazil nuts, 19
breakfast, 45, 58, 63, 72, 81, 85, 93, 102, 116, 124
breathing: aerobics, 20
    and air pollution, 50
    'bellows breath', 94
    curled tongue breaths, 89
    energizing exercises, 59
    Energizing Plan, 91
    natural pain relief, 81
    Stress-busting Plan, 71
    yoga, 21, 22, 23, 104

caffeine, 6, 8–9, 41
    and immune system, 96
    Anti-cellulite Plan, 120
    Decaf Plan, 56–9
    Stress-busting Plan, 68
    Sugar-busting Plan, 63
    and weight gain, 100
calcium, 90, 97, 100, 107
calories, 100, 101, 107, 122
cancer, 9, 74, 82, 121, 122, 125
car travel, 51
carbohydrates, 13, 58, 62, 63
    Energizing Plan, 90–1, 94–5
    Lighten-up Plan, 46, 47
    Stress-busting Plan, 70, 71
carbon monoxide, 9, 50, 52, 82
carpets, pesticides in, 50–1
carrier oils, 34–5
carrots, 19
cellulite, 114–20
chelating foods, 52, 53, 103
chicken, 62, 72
chlorella, 38–9
chlorophyll, 80, 94
chocolate, 47, 64, 124
cholesterol, 19, 74, 124, 125
chromium, 90
cigarettes see smoking
cleaning products, 49, 55
cleansing skin, 110
clothes, 52
clutter, 93

coffee, 8–9, 14, 41, 56, 59, 68, 100
colds, 96, 97
collagen, 108, 109, 112, 114, 115, 120
computers, 52
conjugated linoleic acid (CLA), 101
constipation, 13, 40, 41, 87
cortisol, 66, 92, 101
coughs, 82, 87, 96
cravings: alcohol, 30, 77
    caffeine, 41, 46, 57–8
    cigarettes, 30, 83, 87–9
    sugar, 30, 47, 64
cruciferous vegetables, 18, 80
cypress oil, 36
cysteine, 75, 80

dairy foods, 9, 10, 15, 62, 71, 101, 107
dandelion, 39
Decaf Plan, 56–9
dehydration, 19, 29, 75, 77, 78, 79, 80
depression, 87
diet see food
digestion, 11, 16, 93
    food intolerance, 9, 41, 99, 101
diuretics, 36, 37, 39

Eastern exercise, 21
echinacea, 97, 99
eggs, 19, 80
elastin, 108, 109, 114, 120
electromagnetic fields, 51, 52
elimination diet, 98
Energizing Plan, 90–5
energy, 13, 21, 59, 61, 88
enzymes, 11, 16, 124
essential fatty acids, 112
essential oils:
    aromatherapy, 30, 34–7, 59, 70, 78–9
    baths, 95
    massage, 30, 34–5, 106
    skin care, 111, 120
evening meals, 47, 58, 64, 81, 86, 94–5, 103, 116
exercise, 20–7, 47
    aerobics, 20–1, 94
    and air pollution, 50
    Anti-cellulite Plan, 117–19
    energizing, 59
    Energizing Plan, 94
    and immune system, 97
    and life expectancy, 125
    Stress-busting Plan, 70
    and sugar cravings, 64
    Weight-loss Plan, 104–5, 107

exfoliation, 110
fasting, 13
fat: Anti-cellulite Plan, 114–20
    breakdown of, 20
    fat-burning inhibitors, 100–1
    and longevity, 122
    saturated fats, 10, 15
    weight gain, 100
fat cells: cellulite, 114–15
    toxin storage, 11, 13, 16, 49
fatigue, 70–1, 94, 95
fennel oil, 36
fibre, 13, 19, 40, 41
fish, 62–3
flu, 96, 97
fluid retention, 36, 37, 39, 101, 106
folic acid, 80, 124
food, 15–19
    elimination diet, 98
    food intolerance, 9, 41, 99, 101
    labels, 61
    pesticide residues, 7, 9, 15–16, 100
    see also individual plans
free radicals, 16, 19, 39, 100, 109, 112
    and ageing, 121–2, 123
    and cellulite, 114
    exercise and, 20
    pollution, 10, 48, 52
    sugar and, 60
friends, 125
fruit: alkaline foods, 84
    antioxidants, 115
    juices, 13, 46, 58, 80, 93
    and life expectancy, 123
    pesticide residues, 15–16
    snacks, 46, 47
    top detox foods, 17–19

garlic, 18, 123–4
genetics, and ageing, 121
geranium oil, 36–37
germs, 96–8
ginkgo biloba, 59, 116
ginseng, 70–1
glucose, 90–1
glutathione, 39, 75, 124
glycaemic index, 62, 63
gotu kola, 115, 120
grapefruit oil, 37
green tea, 89, 115, 123
gymnema sylvestre, 64

hair, 109–13
hands, washing, 98
hangovers, 8, 12, 14
    Post-party Hangover Plan, 78–81
    Pre-party Plan, 74–7

happiness, 97
hayfever, 99
head massage, 31
headaches, 41, 57, 59, 67, 78, 79, 81
health, 96–9
health checks, 125
heart: disease, 74, 82, 121, 122
effects of stress, 66, 67
garlic and, 123–4
heat treatments, 29
heavy metals, 9, 17, 19, 38
homeopathy, 81
homocysteine, 124
hormones, 8, 66, 68, 70
horse chestnut, 120

illness, 96–9
immune system, 37, 60, 66, 67, 96–9, 125
inhalations, 34
insomnia, 87
insulin, 61, 65
iodine, 112
iron, 90, 97
irritable bowel syndrome (IBS), 99

juices, 13, 45, 46, 58, 80, 93
juniper oil, 34, 37

kidneys, 11, 16
kiwi fruit, 18
kudzu, 77

laxatives, 40
leafy green vegetables, 80
'leaky gut', 40
lemon oil, 37, 87
lettuce, 71
life expectancy, 121–5
Lighten-up Plan, 44–7
Live Longer Plan, 121–5
liver, 10, 11, 16, 74, 75, 78
lobelia, 88
lunch, 46–7, 58, 63, 70, 81, 85–6, 93, 94, 102–3, 116
lungs, 11, 82
lymphatic system, 11
and cellulite, 114–15
manual lymph drainage, 30, 106
stimulating, 20, 21, 30, 36–7, 98

magnesium, 90, 97, 100–101
mandarin oil, 37
mango and avocado salad, 54
manual lymph drainage, 30, 106
massage, 30–3, 34–5, 106, 109
meat, 10, 15, 123

metabolic rate, 13
migraine, 98–9
milk, 71
milk thistle, 39, 75
minerals, 90
mitochondria, 91, 94
moisturizers, 111
multivitamins, 39–40, 89
muscles: exercise, 94
stretching, 45, 68
tension, 68
toning, 117–19
Weight-loss Plan, 104
yoga, 21

N-Acetyl-Cysteine, 75
neck massage, 31
negative emotions, 97
nicotiana, 88
nicotine, 9, 82–9
Nux Vom, 81

oats, 84
office equipment, 52
oils see essential oils
omega-3 fatty acids, 62
onions, 71
optimism, 125
organic food, 15–16, 50–1, 100
oxygen, 81, 90, 91, 94
oxygen juice, 93

painkillers, 81
parties: Post-party Hangover Plan, 78–81
Pre-party Plan, 74–7
passive smoking, 51, 89
patchouli oil, 37
pessimism, 125
pesticides, 7, 9, 15–16, 48, 50–1, 100
planning, beating stress, 67
plants, 52
pollution, 9–10, 48–55
pose of a child, 79
potassium, 19, 39
pre-menstrual syndrome, 99
probiotics, 40
protein, 46–7, 58, 62, 71, 80, 112, 116
prunes, 18
psyllium husks, 40, 41

rashes, 41
red blood cells, 91, 94, 108, 109
Rescue Remedy, 71
retinol, 120
rheumatoid arthritis, 96, 99
rhinitis, 99
rhodiola, 64
salads, 54
salt, 112
'Salute to the Sun', 69, 92

sandwiches, 54
saturated fats, 10, 15, 122
saunas, 29, 55, 79, 98
scrubs, body, 28
seaweed, 18, 41
selenium, 19
serotonin, 60, 62, 64, 70, 71
side-effects, detoxing, 41
skin: ageing, 109
Anti-cellulite Plan, 114–20
Beauty-boosting Plan, 108–13
body-brushing, 28–9, 92, 120
detoxing side-effects, 41
natural detoxing, 11
sleep, 47, 70–1, 78, 87, 95, 97
smell, sense of, 34
smoking, 7, 9, 10, 29, 39
and ageing, 122
effects on skin, 108
and immune system, 96
passive smoking, 51, 89
Stop Smoking Plan, 82–9
smoothies, 45, 53
snacks, 46, 47, 58, 62–3, 86, 88, 93–4, 102, 103
sodium, 101
soups, 46, 103
steam treatments, 29, 110
stomach: alcohol and, 75, 76
cramps, 41
stress, 10
effects on skin, 109
and immune system, 96, 97
smoking and, 87
Stress-busting Plan, 66–73
stress hormones, 8, 66, 68, 70
and weight gain, 101
yoga and, 21
stretching exercises, 45, 68
sugar, 10, 14, 41, 58, 112, 123
Sugar-busting Plan, 60–5
sulphur, 112
sunlight, 98, 109
sunscreen, 112, 113, 120
supplements, 38–40, 45, 55
sweating, 11, 13, 20, 28, 79

tea, 41, 56, 89, 115, 123
thinking clearly, 87
tiredness, 70–1, 94, 95
toast, 80
tofu, 19, 53
tomatoes, 89
toxins, 8–10
and ageing, 121–2
natural detoxing, 11
toxic overload, 7, 12, 96, 108

traditional detox, 13
triglycerides, 74

ultraviolet rays, 98, 113
urination, increased, 41

vanilla, 47, 64
vegetables: alkaline foods, 84
antioxidants, 115
juices, 13, 46
leafy green vegetables, 80
and life expectancy, 123
pesticide residues, 15–16
top detox foods, 17–19
vegetarian diet, 123
viruses, 97
vitamins, 39–40, 89, 90
vitamin A, 112
vitamin B complex, 68, 75, 76, 80, 90, 93, 97, 109, 112
vitamin C, 39, 75–6, 80, 97, 100, 101, 122
vitamin D, 97, 98
vitamin E, 100
vitamin H, 112
volatile organic compounds (VOCs), 52

waking up, 92
walking, 51–2, 94, 125
water, 19, 29, 41, 58, 77
watercress, 18, 80
Weight-loss Plan, 100–7
wheat, 9, 15, 101, 107
white blood cells, 11, 60, 66, 67, 96, 97, 98
white willow bark, 81
working environment, 52
wrinkles, 108, 109, 121

yoga, 21–7, 68, 69, 79, 89, 104–5, 110

zinc, 76, 90, 97

acknowledgements

A number of people helped with the formation of this book, even though some of them may not have realized it. Over the last 12 years of writing, I have had the privilege of speaking to some of the UK's best nutritionists, who have given me enough of their knowledge to allow me to write this book. Therefore, in no particular order, I would like to (finally) thank Natalie Savona, Antony Haynes, Patrick Holford, Lyndel Costain and Ian 'The Food Doctor' Marber.

I'd also like to thank Robert Tisserand from Tisserand Aromatherapy and Glenda Taylor from Cariad for all the knowledge they have given me on aromatherapy. As for fitness, the list is endless, but Dean Hodgkin, Luke Wilkins, Giles Smith, Joseph Sgro all deserve special mention. Huge thanks go to the team at Platinum Health Club in Milford, Auckland, New Zealand, especially Fay Todd, who compiled, checked and rechecked all the yoga programmes in the book. Acupuncturist Yuki Umiguchi also deserves thanks for her tips on acupuncture and acupressure, while beauty experts John Prothero at Michaeljohn Hair Salon in Mayfair, Sally Penford from the International Dermal Institute and make-up artist/beauty writer Virginia Nichols taught me a great deal.

While I carried out the majority of the research for the book myself, there are two excellent books I must credit. They are *The Detox Diet* by Paula Baillie Hamilton (Penguin, 2002) and *The Cellulite Solution* by Elisabeth Dancey (Hodder and Stoughton, 1996).

At Hamlyn, I have to thank Nicola Hill for coming up with the idea and sparking my interest, and Jane Birch for making sense of it all and turning it into what you see today.

Personal thanks go to commissioning editors Andrew Fleming, Simone Cave and Ursula Kenny, who put up with me disappearing for a month at a time to get things started and finished; to Tim, who listened to endless 'I'm never going to get this finished' conversations and answered them all with another cup of tea; and to my mum and dad, Sandra and Martin, who supported me when 'writing for a living' was just a dream.

Helen Foster

Photographic acknowledgements

Getty Images 4, 20, 21, 50, 72, 73, 88, 91 bottom right/Roy Botterell 40/Alain Daussin 97/Britt Erlanson 14 bottom right, 92 top right/Chris Everard 14 top left/Carol Ford 29, 103/J.P. Fruchet 6/Rob Gage 12/Nello Giambi 48/Larry Dale Gordon 49/Diana Healey 100/Edward Holub 109 top left/Richard Kolker 82/Uwe Krejci 44/Romilly Lockyear 66/Rita Maas 13/David Madison 104/Megumi Miyatake 87/Giuseppe Molteni 39/David Oliver 52 top left/Lee Page 91 top left/Joe Polillio 38/Darren Robb 121/Ralf Schultheiss 45 **Octopus Publishing Group Limited**/Jean Cazals 8, 78/Stephen Conroy 93, 95 bottom right, 116/Jerry Harpur 70/Jeremy Hopley 76 bottom left, 92 bottom left/David Jordan 19, 46, 60, 62, 124/Sandra Lane 17 top, 17 bottom, 36, 37, 65 top right, 85 top, 123 right/Gary Latham 65 bottom left/William Lingwood 1, 18, 52 bottom right, 54 bottom right, 54 bottom left/Neil Mersh 79 top left/Peter Myers 68/Sean Myers 80 top, 86 top/Peter Pugh-Cook 22 top, 22 centre, 22 bottom, 23, 24 top, 24 bottom, 25 right, 25 top left, 25 bottom left, 26 top, 26 bottom, 27 top, 27 centre, 27 bottom right, 27 bottom left, 31 centre left, 31 top right, 31 bottom right, 32 centre left, 32 top right, 32 bottom right, 33 top left, 33 top right, 33 bottom left, 35, 105 top right, 105 centre right, 105 top left, 105 centre left, 105 top right, 117 bottom right, 117 bottom left, 118 top left, 118 bottom right, 118 bottom left, 119 top left, 119 bottom right, 119 bottom left/William Reavell 15, 16, 34, 53, 64, 74, 76 bottom right, 77, 83, 85 bottom, 90, 95 centre right, 102, 111 bottom left, 123 left/Gareth Sambidge 67/Simon Smith 10, 61/Karen Thomas 85 centre/Ian Wallace 3, 28, 30, 42, 55, 57, 69 top left, 69 centre, 69 top right, 69 bottom right, 69 bottom left, 71, 79 bottom right, 89, 94, 106, 107, 108, 109 bottom right, 110, 111 bottom right, 113, 114, 115/Philip Webb 86 bottom

Executive Editor Nicola Hill
Editor Joss Waterfall
Executive Art Editor Jo MacGregor
Designer Ruth Hope
Picture Researcher Christine Junemann

Senior Production Controller Jo Sim
Special Photography Peter Pugh-Cook
Exercise Consultant Chrissie Gallagher-Mundy
Massage Consultant Natalie McDonnell